Clinical Skills and Examination

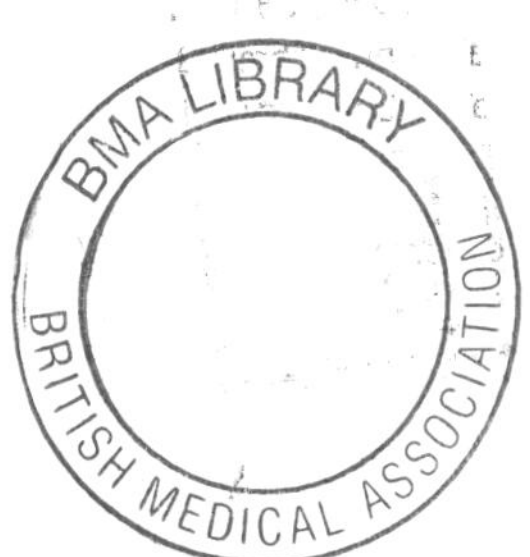

Commissioning Editor: Elizabeth Johnston
Production Editor: Cathryn Gates
Development Editor: Laura Quigley
Editorial Assistant: Madeleine Hurd

Clinical Skills and Examination

THE CORE CURRICULUM

by

Robert Turner, MD, FRCP
The late Professor of Medicine and
Director of the Diabetes Research Laboratories
University of Oxford
Oxford, UK

Brian John Angus, DTM&H, MD, FRCP
Clinical Tutor in Medicine and
Consultant Physician
Nuffield Department of Medicine
John Radcliffe Hospital
Oxford, UK

Ashok Handa, FRCS, FRSC (Ed)
Clinical Tutor in Surgery and
Consultant Surgeon
Nuffield Department of Surgery
John Radcliffe Hospital
Oxford, UK

Chris Hatton, FRCP, FRCPath
Consultant Haematologist
Department of Haematology
John Radcliffe Hospital
Oxford, UK

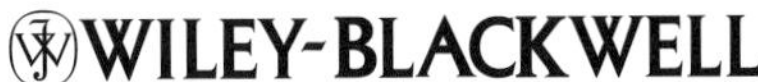

A John Wiley & Sons, Ltd., Publication

Blackwell Publishing was acquired by John Wiley & Sons in February 2007. Blackwell's publishing program has been merged with Wiley's global Scientific, Technical and Medical business to form Wiley-Blackwell.

Registered office: John Wiley & Sons Ltd, The Atrium, Southern Gate, Chichester, West Sussex, PO19 8SQ, UK

Editorial offices: 9600 Garsington Road, Oxford, OX4 2DQ, UK
The Atrium, Southern Gate, Chichester, West Sussex, PO19 8SQ, UK
111 River Street, Hoboken, NJ 07030-5774, USA

For details of our global editorial offices, for customer services and for information about how to apply for permission to reuse the copyright material in this book please see our website at www.wiley.com/wiley-blackwell

Library of Congress Cataloging-in-Publication Data

Clinical skills and examination : the core curriculum / by Robert Turner . . . [et al.]. – 5th ed.
p. ; cm.
Rev. ed. of: Lecture notes on clinical skills / Roger Blackwood. 4th ed. 2003.
Includes bibliographical references.
ISBN 978-1-4051-5751-3
1. Medical history taking–Handbooks, manuals, etc. 2. Physical diagnosis–Handbooks, manuals, etc. I. Turner, Robert (Robert Charles), 1938– II. Blackwood, Roger. Lecture notes on clinical skills.
[DNLM: 1. Medical History Taking–Handbooks. 2. Physical Examination–Handbooks. WB 39 C6416 2009]
RC65.T87 2009
616.07′51–dc22

2008039509

ISBN: 9781405157513

A catalogue record for this book is available from the British Library.

Set in 8 on 11 pt Syntax by SNP Best-set Typesetter Ltd., Hong Kong
Printed and bound in Singapore by Markono Print Media Pte Ltd

3 2015

Contents

SECTION I

History and examination

CHAPTER 1

History taking

General procedures

Approaching the patient

- **Look the part of a doctor and put the patient at ease. Be confident and quietly friendly.**
- **Greet the patient politely: 'Good morning, Mr Smith'.**
- **Shake the patient's hand or place your hand on their hand if they are ill.**
- **State your name and that you are a medical student.**
- **Make sure the patient is comfortable.**
- **Explain that you wish to ask the patient some questions to find out what happened to them.**

  Inform the patient how long you are likely to take and what to expect. For example, after discussing what has happened to the patient, you would like to examine them. Most patients are very happy to have someone to chat to but if they do not then don't take it personally.

- **Confirm the patient's name, age and occupation (if retired, then previous occupation).**

Usual sequence of events

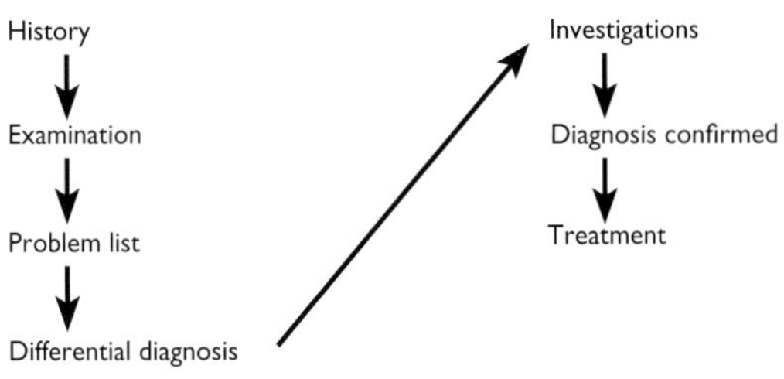

Clinical Skills and Examination: The Core Curriculum. By R Turner, B Angus, A Handa, C Hatton. ©2009 Blackwell Publishing, ISBN: 9781405157513.

Importance of the history

- It identifies:
  - what has happened
  - the personality of the patient
  - how the illness has affected them and their family
  - any specific anxieties
  - the physical and social environment.
- It establishes the physician–patient relationship.
- It often suggests the diagnosis.

- **Find the principal symptoms or symptom with an open question. Ask:**
  - **'What has the problem been?'**
  - **'What made you go to the doctor?'**

  Avoid:
  - 'What's wrong?' or 'What brought you here?'
- **Let the patient tell their story in their own words as much as possible.**

  At first listen and then take discreet notes as they talk. When learning to take a history there can be a tendency to ask too many questions in the first 2 minutes. After asking the first question you should normally allow the patient to talk uninterrupted for up to 2 minutes.

  Do not worry if the story is not entirely clear, or if you do not think the information being given is of diagnostic significance. If you interrupt too early, you run the risk of overlooking an important symptom or anxiety.

  - **You will be learning about what the patient thinks is important.**
  - **You have the opportunity to judge how you are going to proceed.**

  Different patients give histories in very different ways. Some patients will need to be encouraged to enlarge on their answers to your questions; with other patients you may need to ask specific questions and interrupt in order to prevent too rambling a history. Think consciously about the approach you will adopt. If you need to interrupt the patient, do so clearly and decisively.

- **Try, if feasible, to conduct a conversation rather than an interrogation, following the patient's train of thoughts.**

You will usually need to ask follow-up questions on the main symptoms to obtain a full understanding of what they were and of the chain of events. Try to note down the main points and then explore those.

- **Obtain a full description of the patient's principal complaints.**
- **Enquire about the sequence of symptoms and events.**

Beware pseudomedical terms and jargon, e.g. 'gastric flu'—enquire what happened.

- **Do not ask leading questions at first.**

A central aim in taking the history is to understand the patient's symptoms from their point of view. It is important not to colour the patient's history with your own expectations. For example, do not ask a patient whom you suspect might be thyrotoxic: 'Do you find hot weather uncomfortable?' This invites the answer 'Yes' and then a positive answer becomes of little diagnostic value. Ask the open question: 'Do you particularly dislike either hot or cold weather?'

- **Be sensitive to a patient's mood and non-verbal responses.**

For example, hesitancy in revealing emotional content. Remember the importance of non-verbal communication.

- **Be understanding, receptive and matter-of-fact without excessive sympathy.**
- **Rarely show surprise or reproach.**
- **Clarify symptoms and obtain a problem list.** When the patient has finished describing the symptom or symptoms:
  - **briefly summarise the symptoms**
  - **ask whether there are any other main problems.**

For example, say, 'You have mentioned two problems: pain on the left side of your tummy, and loose motions over the past 6 weeks. Before we talk about those in more detail, are there any other problems I should know about?'

Usual sequence of history

- nature of principal complaints, e.g. chest pain, poor home circumstances
- history of present complaint—details of current illness
- enquiry of other symptoms (see Functional enquiry below)
- past history
- drug history including allergies and over the counter medication
- family history
- personal and social history, including travel and animal contact

- If one's initial enquiries make it apparent that one section is of more importance than usual (e.g. previous relevant illnesses or operation), then relevant enquiries can be brought forward to an earlier stage in the history (e.g. past history after finding principal complaints).

History of present illness

- **Start your written history with a single sentence** summing up what your patient is complaining of. It should be like the banner headline of a newspaper. For example:

  c/o chest pain for 6 months.

- **Determine the chronology of the illness by asking:**
  - 'How and when did your illness begin?' or
  - 'When did you first notice anything wrong?' or
  - 'When did you last feel completely well?'
- **Begin by stating when the patient was last perfectly well.** Describe symptoms in **chronological order of onset**.

  Both the **date of onset** and the **length of time** prior to admission should be recorded. Symptoms should never be dated by the day of the week as this later becomes meaningless.

- **Obtain a detailed description of each symptom by asking:**
  - 'Tell me what the pain was like', for example. Make sure you ask about all symptoms, whether they seem relevant or not.
- **With all symptoms obtain the following details:**
  - **duration**
  - **onset—sudden or gradual**
  - **what has happened since:**
    - **constant or periodic**
    - **frequency**
    - **getting worse or better**
  - **precipitating or relieving factors**
  - **associated symptoms.**
- **If pain is a symptom, also determine the following:**
  - **site**
  - **radiation**
    - **character**, e.g. ache, pressure, shooting, stabbing, dull
    - **severity**, e.g. 'Did it interfere with what you were doing? Does it keep you awake?'
  - have you ever had this pain before?
  - is the pain associated with nausea, sweating, e.g. angina?

Avoid technical language when describing a patient's history. Do not say 'the patient complained of melaena', rather: 'the patient complained of passing loose, black, tarry motions'.

Students often find the mnemonic SOCRATES useful: **S**ite, **O**nset, **C**haracter, **R**adiation, **A**lleviating factors/ **A**ssociated symptoms, **T**iming (duration, frequency), **E**xacerbating factors, **S**everity.

Supplementary history

When patients are unable to give an adequate or reliable history, the necessary information must be obtained from friends, relations or carers. A history from a person who has witnessed a sudden event is often helpful.

Accordingly, the student should arrange with the F1 doctor to be present when the relatives or witnesses are interviewed. This is particularly important with patients suffering from disease of the central nervous system. The date and source of such information should be written in the notes.

When necessary, arrange for an interpreter. This can be done via local authorities. Be careful about using family members to translate.

Make use of the GP's letter and contact the GP if necessary.

Functional enquiry

This is a checklist of symptoms not already discovered. Do not ask questions already covered in establishing the principal symptoms. This list may detect other symptoms.

- **Modify your questioning according to the nature of the suspected disease, available time and circumstances.**

If during the functional enquiry a positive answer is obtained, full details must be elicited. Asterisks (*) denote questions which must nearly always be asked.

General questions

- Ask about the following points.
  - ***Appetite**: 'What is your appetite like? Do you feel like eating?'
  - ***Weight**: 'Have you lost or gained weight recently?' This is a crucially important question!
  - ***General wellbeing**: 'Do you feel well in yourself?'
  - **Fatigue**: 'Are you more or less tired than you used to be?'
  - **Fever or chills**: 'Have you felt hot or cold? Have you shivered?'
  - **Night sweats**: 'Have you noticed any sweating at night or any other time? Enough to soak the bedclothes?'
  - **Aches or pains**.

- **Rash**: 'Have you had any rash recently? Does it itch?'
- **Lumps and bumps**.

Cardiovascular and respiratory system

- Ask about the following points.
  - ***Chest pain**: 'Have you recently had any pain or discomfort in the chest?'

The most common causes of chest pain are:

Ischaemic heart disease: severe constricting, central chest pain radiating to the neck, jaw and left arm.

Angina is this pain precipitated by exercise or emotion; relieved by rest.

In a *myocardial infarction* the pain may come on at rest, be more severe and last hours.

Pleuritic pain: sharp, localised pain, usually lateral; worse on deep inspiration or cough.

Anxiety or panic attacks are a very common cause of chest pain. Enquire about circumstances that bring on an attack.

- ***Shortness of breath**: 'Are you breathless at any time?'

Breathlessness (*dyspnoea*) and chest pain must be accurately described. The degree of exercise that brings on the symptoms must be noted (e.g. climbing one flight of stairs, after 0.5 km (1/4 mile) walk).

- **Shortness of breath on lying flat** (*orthopnoea*): 'Do you get breathless in bed? Can you lie flat? What do you do then? Does it get worse or better on sitting up? How many pillows do you use? Can you sleep without them?'
- **Waking up breathless**: 'Do you wake at night with any symptoms? Do you gasp for breath? What do you do then?'

Orthopnoea (breathless when lying flat) and *paroxysmal nocturnal dyspnoea* (suddenly waking up breathless, relieved on sitting up) are features of *left heart failure*.

- ***Ankle swelling**.

Common in *congestive cardiac failure* (*right heart failure*).

- **Palpitations**: 'Are you aware of your heart beating?'

Palpitations may be:
- single thumps (*ectopics*)
- slow or fast
- regular or irregular.

Ask the patient to tap them out.
Paroxysmal tachycardia (sudden attacks of palpitations) usually starts and finishes abruptly.

- ***Cough**: 'Do you have a cough? Is it a dry cough or do you cough up sputum? When do you cough?'
- **Sputum**: 'What colour is your sputum? How much do you cough up?'

Green sputum usually indicates an *acute chest infection*. Clear sputum daily during winter months suggests *chronic bronchitis*. Frothy sputum suggests *left heart failure*.

- ***Blood in sputum** (*haemoptysis*): 'Have you coughed up blood?'

Haemoptysis must be taken very seriously. Causes include:
carcinoma of bronchus
pulmonary embolism
mitral stenosis
tuberculosis
bronchiectasis.

- **Black-outs** (*syncope*): 'Have you had any black-outs or faints? Did you feel light-headed or did the room go round? Did you lose consciousness? Did you have any warning? Can you remember what happened?'
- ***Smoking**: 'Do you smoke? How many cigarettes do you smoke?'

Gastrointestinal system

- Ask about the following points.
  - **Mouth ulcers.**
  - **Nausea**: 'Are there times when you feel sick?'

- **Vomiting**: 'Have you vomited? What is it like?'

'Coffee grounds' vomit suggests altered blood.
Old food suggests *pyloric stenosis*.
If blood, what colour is it—dark or bright red?

- **Difficulty in swallowing** (*dysphagia*): 'Do you have difficulty swallowing? Where does it stick?'

For solids: often organic obstruction.
For fluids: often neurological or psychological.

- **Indigestion**: 'Do you have any discomfort in your stomach after eating?'
- **Abdominal pain**: 'Where is the pain? How is it connected to meals or opening your bowels? What relieves the pain?'
- **Bowel habit**: 'Is your bowel habit regular? How many times do you open your bowels per day? Do you have to open your bowels at night?' (*often a sign of true pathology*).

If *diarrhoea* is suggested, the number of motions per day and their nature (blood? pus? mucus? slime?) must be established.

'What are your motions like?' The stools may be pale, bulky and float (fat in stool—*steatorrhoea*) or tarry from digested blood (*melaena*—usually from upper gastrointestinal tract).

Bright blood on the surface of a motion may be from *haemorrhoids*, whereas blood in a stool may signify *cancer* or *inflammatory bowel disease*.

Tenesmus is a feeling of incomplete evacuation and is highly suspicious of a colonic polyp or malignancy.

- **Jaundice**: 'Have you noticed any yellowing of the eyes? Is your urine dark? Are your stools pale? What tablets have you been taking recently? Have you had any recent injections or transfusions? Have you been abroad recently? How much alcohol do you drink?'

Jaundice may be:

- **obstructive** (dark urine, pale stools) from: *carcinoma of the head of the pancreas* or *gallstones*

- **hepatocellular** (dark urine, pale stools may develop) from:
  ethanol (*cirrhosis*)
  intravenous drug abuse, tattoos, unprotected sex or transfusions (*viral hepatitis*)
  drug reactions or infections (travel abroad, *viral hepatitis, malaria* or *amoebae*)
- **haemolytic** (unconjugated bilirubin is bound to albumin and is not secreted in the urine).

Genitourinary system

- Ask about the following points.
  - **Dysuria**: pain on passing urine, usually burning (*often a sign of infection*).
  - **Loin pain**: 'Any pain in your back?'

Pain in the loins suggests *pyelonephritis* or *renal colic*.

- ***Urine**: 'Are your waterworks all right? Do you pass a lot of water at night? Do you have any difficulty passing water? Is there blood in your water?'—*haematuria*.

Polyuria and *nocturia* occur in *diabetes*.

Prostatism results in slow onset of urination (*hesitancy*), a poor stream and terminal dribbling.

- **Sex**: 'Any problems with intercourse or making love?' **If appropriate** ask about last sexual partner, whether regular or casual, oral, vaginal or anal sex. Homosexual contact? Risk factors for HIV should be explored where appropriate.
- ***Menstruation**: 'Any problems with your periods? Do you bleed heavily? Do you bleed between periods?'

Vaginal bleeding between periods or after the menopause raises the possibility of *cervical* or *uterine cancer*.

- **Vaginal or penile discharge**.
- **Menstrual cycle**: last menstrual period (LMP) and abnormal vaginal bleeding:

- *inter-menstrual bleeding*
- *post-menopausal bleeding*
- *post-coital bleeding.*

- **Pain on intercourse** (*dyspareunia*) and whether this is superficial or deep.

Nervous system

- Ask about the following points.
  - ***Headache**: 'Do you have any headaches? Where are they, when do you get headaches?'

For example, early morning headaches may suggest *raised intracranial pressure—tumour.*

Are the headaches associated with flashing lights (*migraine*) or scalp tenderness (*polymyalgia rheumatica*)?

- **Vision**: 'Do you have any blurred or double vision?'
- **Hearing**: ask about tinnitus, deafness and exposure to noise.
- **Dizziness**: 'Do you have any dizziness or episodes when the world goes round (*vertigo*)?'

Dizziness with light-headed symptoms, when sudden in onset, may be *cardiac* (enquire about palpitations). When slow, onset may be *vasovagal 'fainting'* or an *internal haemorrhage*.

Vertigo may be from *ear disease* (enquire about deafness, earache or discharge) or *brainstem dysfunction*.

- **Unsteady gait**: 'Any difficulty walking or running?'
- **Weakness**: 'Do your arms or legs feel weak?'
- **Numbness** or increased sensation: 'Any patches of numbness?'
- **Pins and needles**.
- **Sphincter disturbance**: 'Any difficulties holding your water/bowels?' (*a very important sign of spinal cord compression*).
- **Fits or faints**: 'Have you had any funny turns?'

The following details should be sought from the patient and any observer:

- **duration**
- **frequency** and length of attacks
- **time of attacks**, e.g. if standing, at night
- **mode of onset and termination**, e.g. post-ictal phase
- **premonition or aura**, light-headed or vertigo
- **biting of tongue, loss of sphincter control, injury, etc.**

Grand mal epilepsy classically produces sudden unconsciousness without any warning and on waking the patient feels drowsy with a headache and sore tongue, and has been incontinent.

Mental state

- Ask about the following points.
  - **Depression**: 'How is your mood? Happy or sad? If depressed, how bad? Have you lost interest in things? Can you still enjoy things? How do you feel about the future?'
    'Has anything happened in your life to make you depressed? Do you feel guilty about anything?'
    If the patient appears depressed: 'Have you ever thought of suicide? How long have you felt like this? Is there a specific problem? Have you felt like this before?'
  - **Active periods**: 'Do you have periods in which you are particularly active?'

Susceptibility to depression may be a personality trait. In *bipolar depression*, swings to *mania* (excess activity, rapid speech and excitable mood) can recur. Enquire about interest, concentration, irritability, sleep difficulties.

- **Anxiety**:
  - 'Have you worried a lot recently? Do you get anxious? In what situations? Are there any situations you avoid because you feel anxious?'
  - 'Do you worry about your health? Any worries in your job or with your family? Any financial worries?'
  - 'Do you have panic attacks? What happens?'
- **Sleep**: 'Any difficulties sleeping? Do you have difficulty getting to sleep? Do you wake early?'

Difficulties of sleep are commonly associated with depression or anxiety.

A more complete assessment of mental state is given in Chapter 6.

The eye

- Ask about the following points.
  - **Eye pain, photophobia or redness**: 'Have your eyes been red, uncomfortable or painful?'
  - Painful red eye, particularly with photophobia, may be serious and due to:

iritis (ankylosing spondylitis, Reiter's disease, sarcoid, Behçet's disease)
scleritis (systemic vasculitis)
corneal ulcer
acute glaucoma
photophobia may be a sign of meningitis.

  - Painless red eye may be:

episcleritis
temporary and of no consequence
systemic vasculitis.

  - Sticky red eye may be *conjunctivitis* (usually infective).
  - Itchy eye may be *allergic*, e.g. *hayfever.*
  - Gritty eye may be dry (sicca or *Sjögren's syndrome*).
  - **Clarity of vision**: 'Has your vision been blurred?'
    - Blurring of vision for either near or distance alone may be an error of focus, helped by spectacles.
    - Loss of central vision (or of top or bottom half) in one eye may be due to a *retinal* or *optic nerve disorder*.
    - Transient complete blindness in one eye lasting for minutes—*amaurosis fugax* (fleeting blindness)—suggests retinal arterial blockage from embolus, may be from *carotid atheroma* (listen for bruit) or may have a cardiac source.

- Subtle difficulties with vision, difficulty reading—problems at the chiasm, or visual path behind it:

complete *bitemporal hemianopia—tumour* pressure on chiasm

homonymous hemianopia: *posterior cerebral* or *optic radiation lesion*—usually *infarct* or *tumour;* rarely complains of 'half vision', but may have difficulty reading.

- **Diplopia**: 'Have you ever had double vision?'

Diplopia may be due to:

- *lesion* of the motor cranial nerves III, IV or VI
- *third-nerve palsy*
  causes double vision in all directions
  often with dilatation of the pupil and ptosis
  the eye hangs 'down and out'
- *fourth-nerve palsy*
  causes doubling looking down and in (as when reading) with images separated horizontally and vertically and tilted (not parallel)
- *sixth-nerve palsy*
  causes horizontal, level and parallel doubling
  worse on looking to the affected side
- *muscular disorder*
  e.g. thyroid-related (see below)
  myasthenia gravis (weakness after prolonged muscle use, antibodies to nerve end-plates).

Locomotor system

- Ask about the following points.
  - **Pain, stiffness, or swelling of joints**: 'When and how did it start? Have you injured the joint?'

There are innumerable causes of *arthritis* (painful, swollen, tender joints) and *arthralgia* (painful joints). Patients may incorrectly attribute a problem to some injury.

Osteoarthritis is a joint 'wearing out', and is often asymmetric, involving weight-bearing joints such as the hip or knee. Exercise makes the joint pain worse.

Rheumatoid arthritis is a generalised autoimmune disease with symmetrical involvement. In the hands, fusiform swelling of the interphalangeal joints is accompanied by swollen metacarpophalangeal joints. Large joints are often affected. Stiffness is worse after rest, e.g. on waking, and improves with use.

Gout usually involves a single joint, such as the first metatarsophalangeal joint, but can lead to gross hand involvement with asymmetric uric acid lumps (*tophi*) by some joints, and in the tips of the ears.

Septic arthritis: this is important not to miss—a single, hot painful joint.

- **Functional disability**: 'How far can you walk? Can you walk upstairs? Is any particular movement difficult? Can you dress yourself? How long does it take? Can you work? Can you write?'

Thyroid disease

- Ask about the following points.
  - **Weight change**.
  - **Reaction to the weather**: 'Do you dislike the hot or cold weather?'
  - **Irritability**: 'Are you more or less irritable compared with a few years ago?'
  - **Diarrhoea/constipation**.
  - **Palpitations**.
  - **Dry skin or greasy hair**: 'Is your skin dry or greasy? Is your hair dry or greasy?'
  - **Depression**: 'How has your mood been?'
  - **Croaky voice**.

Hypothyroid patients put on weight without increase in appetite, dislike cold weather, have dry skin and thin, dry hair, a puffy face, a croaky voice, are usually calm and may be depressed.

Hyperthyroid patients may lose weight despite eating more, dislike hot weather, perspire excessively, have palpitations, a tremor, and may be agitated and tearful. Young people have predominantly nervous and heat intolerance symptoms, whereas old people tend to present with cardiac symptoms.

Past history

- **All previous illnesses or operations**, whether apparently important or not, must be included.

For instance, a casually mentioned attack of influenza or chill may have been a manifestation of an occult infection. Try to establish a date.

For operations try to get an approximate date (which year or how many years ago), name of surgeon and institution where it was carried out.

- The importance of a past illness may be gained by finding out **how long the patient was in bed or off work.**
- **Complications of any previous illnesses** should be carefully enquired into and, here, leading questions are sometimes necessary.

General questions

- Ask about the following.
  - **'Have you had any serious illnesses?'**
  - **'Have you had any emotional or nervous problems?'**
  - **'Have you had any operations or admissions to hospital?'**
  - **'Have you ever:**
    - **had myocardial infarction (heart attack), jaundice (yellowing of the eyes), TB, hypertension (high blood pressure), rheumatic fever, epilepsy, anaemia, diabetes, syncope (faints)? (remember MJTHREADS)**
    - **had allergies?'**
  - **'Have any medicines ever upset you?'**

Allergic responses to drugs may include an itchy rash, vomiting, diarrhoea or severe illness, including jaundice. Many patients claim to be allergic but are not, e.g. GI upset with antibioics. An accurate description of the supposed allergic episodes is important.

  - Additional questions can be asked:
    - if the patient has high blood pressure, ask about kidney problems, or if relatives have kidney disease
    - if a possible heart attack, ask about hypertension, diabetes, diet, smoking, family history of heart disease

- if the patient's history suggests cardiac failure, you must ask if they have had *rheumatic fever*.

Patients have often had examinations for life insurance or the armed forces.

Family history

The family history gives clues to possible predisposition to illness (e.g. heart attacks) **and whether a patient may be particularly anxious about a certain disease** (e.g. mother died of cancer). Death certificates and patient knowledge are often inaccurate. Patients may be reluctant to talk about relatives' illnesses if they were mental diseases, epilepsy or cancer.

General questions

- Ask about the following.
  - '**Are your parents alive?** Are they fit and well? What did your parents die from?'
  - '**Have you any brothers or sisters?** Are they fit and well?'
  - '**Do you have any children?** Are they fit and well?'
  - '**Is there any history of:**
    - **heart trouble?**
    - **diabetes?**
    - **high blood pressure in the family?'**

These questions can be varied to take account of the patient's major complaint.

Personal and social history

One needs to find out what kind of person the patient is, what their home circumstances are and how their illness has affected them and their family. Your aim is to understand the patient's illness in the context of their personality and their home environment.

Can they convalesce satisfactorily at home and at what stage? What are the consequences of their illness? Will advice, information and help be needed? An interview with a relative or friend may be very helpful.

General questions

- Ask about the following.
  - **Marital status**: 'Are you in a relationship?' Find out whether the patient is married or in a partnership and whether they have any children.
  - **Family**: 'Is everything alright at home? Do you have any family problems?'

It **may be appropriate** to ask: 'Is your relationship all right? Is sex all right?' Problems may arise from physical or emotional reasons, and the patient may appreciate an opportunity to discuss worries.

  - **Accommodation**: 'Where do you live? Can you normally manage at home? Is the toilet downstairs or upstairs? Do you cook for yourself at home? Who gets in the shopping?'
  - **Job**: 'What is your job? Could you tell me exactly what you do? Will your illness affect your work?'
  - **Hobbies**: 'What do you do in your spare time?'
  - **Alcohol**: 'How much alcohol do you drink in a week?' The Department of Health advises that men should not drink more than 3–4 units of alcohol per day (28 per week), and women should drink no more than 2–3 units of alcohol per day (21 per week). If there is a suspicion of a drinking problem the CAGE questions are useful to identify problems. 'Have you ever felt you should CUT DOWN on your drinking? Have people ANNOYED you by criticising your drinking? Have you ever felt bad or GUILTY about your drinking? Have you ever had a drink first thing in the morning (as an 'EYE OPENER') to steady your nerves or get rid of a hangover?'
  - **Smoking**: 'Do you smoke? Have you ever smoked? (Remember patients often 'give up' on admission to hospital!) Why did you give up? How many cigarettes, cigars or pipefuls of tobacco do you smoke a day?'

This is particularly relevant for heart or chest disease, but must always be asked.

- **Drugs**: 'Have you ever taken any recreational drugs? Have you ever injected drugs? Have you ever shared needles?'
- **Overseas travel**: 'Have you travelled abroad? Especially to exotic areas within the past month.'
- **Prescribed medications**: 'What pills, tablets or medicines are you taking at the moment? Have you taken any other pills in the past few months?'

This is an extremely important question. A complete list of all drugs and doses must be obtained.

If relevant, ask about any pets, animal contact, previous or present exposure during working to coal dust, asbestos, etc.

The patient's ideas, concerns and expectations

Make sure that you understand the patient's main ideas, concerns and expectations. Either now, or after examining the patient, ask for example:

- **What do you think is wrong with you?**
- **What are you expecting to happen to you while you are in hospital?**
- **Is there something particular you would like us to do?**
- **Have you any questions?**

The patient's main concerns may not be your main concerns. The patient may have quite different expectations of the hospital admission, or outpatient appointment, from what you assume. If you fail to address the patient's concerns they are likely to be dissatisfied, leading to difficult doctor–patient relationships and non-compliance.

Strategy

Having taken the history, you should:

- have some idea of possible diagnoses
- have made an assessment of the patient as a person
- know which systems you wish to concentrate on when examining the patient.

Further relevant questions may arise from abnormalities found on examination or investigation.

Recently some proformas have been developed to enable rapid and focused questions to be asked so that appropriate treatment is not delayed. For example, a care pathway for thrombolysis in patients with suspected heart attacks, a clerk-in sheet for patients with gastrointestinal bleeding containing a Rockall score or a surgical clerk-in sheet. It is worth reviewing these to show which questions are crucial. See examples below.

Specimen history

Date and time of examination in margin
Mr John Smith.
Aged 52. Machine operator. Oxford.
c/o severe chest pain for 2 hours.

History of present illness

- Perfectly well until 6 months ago.
- Began to notice central, dull chest ache, occasionally felt in the jaw, coming on when walking about 1 km (1/2 mile), worse when going uphill and worse in cold weather. When he stopped, the pain went off after 2 minutes.
- Glyceryl trinitrate spray relieved the pain rapidly.
- Last month the pain came on with less exercise after 100 yards.
- Today at 10 am, while sitting at work, the chest pain came on without provocation. It was the worst pain he had ever experienced in his life and he thought he was going to die.
- The pain was central, crushing in nature, radiating to the left arm and neck and with it a feeling of nausea and sweating. The patient was rushed to hospital where he received an intravenous injection of diamorphine, which rapidly relieved the pain, and intravenous streptokinase. An electrocardiogram confirmed a myocardial infarction and the patient was admitted to the coronary care unit.
- The patient had noticed very mild breathlessness on exertion for 3 months, but had not experienced

palpitations, dizziness, breathlessness on lying flat, ankle swelling or coughing. On one occasion, however, 2 weeks ago, the patient had woken with a suffocating feeling and had had to sit on the edge of the bed and subsequently open the bedroom window in order to get his breath. This had not recurred and he did not report it to his doctor.

Functional enquiry

Respiratory system (RS):

- morning cough over the last 3–4 winters with production of a small amount of clear sputum
- no haemoptysis

Gastrointestinal (GI):

- occasional mild indigestion
- bowels regular
- appetite normal
- no other abnormalities

Genitourinary (GU):

- no difficulties with micturition
- normal sex life

Nervous system (NS):

- infrequent frontal headaches at the end of a hectic day
- otherwise no abnormalities
- no psychiatric symptoms

Past medical history

Fifteen years ago, appendicectomy. No complications.
No other operations or serious illnesses.
No history of rheumatic fever, nephritis or hypertension.
Never been abroad.

Family history

Father died aged 73—'heart attack'.
Mother died aged 71—'cancer'.
Two brothers fit and well (aged 48 and 46).
Two sons (aged 23, 25), both fit and well.
No family history of diabetes or hypertension.

Personal and social history

Happy both at work and home. Both sons married and living in Oxford. Wife works as an office cleaner. No financial difficulties.

Smokes 20 cigarettes per day. Two pints of beer on Saturdays only.

Patient always worked as machine operator since leaving school except for 2 years in Hong Kong, where he had no illness.

Medication

Other than glyceryl trinitrate spray, no drugs currently being taken. No allergies.

Signed with name printed and designation (e.g. Medical Student).

CHAPTER 2
General examination

The initial assessment of the patient will have been made while taking a history. The **general appearance of the patient** is the first observation, and thereafter the order of examination will vary.

The system to which the presenting symptoms refer is often examined first. Otherwise devise your own routine, examining each part of the body in turn, covering all systems. An example is:

- **general appearance**
- **alertness, mood, general behaviour**
- **hands and nails**
- **radial pulse and blood pressure**
- **axillary nodes**
- **cervical lymph nodes**
- **facies, eyes, tongue**
- **jugular venous pressure**
- **heart, breasts**
- **respiratory system**
- **spine (while patient is sitting forward)**
- **abdomen, including femoral pulses**
- **legs**
- **nervous system, including fundi**
- **rectal or pelvic examination**
- **gait**.

Whichever part of the body one is examining, one should always use the same routine:

1 **Inspection.**

2 **Palpation.**

Clinical Skills and Examination: The Core Curriculum. By R Turner, B Angus, A Handa, C Hatton. ©2009 Blackwell Publishing, ISBN: 9781405157513.

3 **Percussion.**
4 **Auscultation.**

General inspection

The beginning of the examination is a careful observation of the patient as a whole. Step back from the patient and tell them that you are going to look at them. Note the following:

- **Does the patient look ill?**
  - what age do they look?
  - febrile, dehydrated
  - alert, confused, drowsy
  - cooperative, happy, sad, resentful
  - fat, muscular, wasted
  - in pain or distressed.

Hands

Note the following.

- **Temperature:**
  - unduly cold hands—? *low cardiac output*
  - unduly warm hands—? *high-output state*, e.g. *thyrotoxicosis, sepsis*
  - cold and sweaty—? anxiety or other causes of *sympathetic overreactivity*, e.g. *hypoglycaemia*.
- **Peripheral cyanosis.**
- **Raynaud's** (Figure 2.1).
- **Nicotine staining.**
- **Nails:**
  - bitten
  - leukonychia—white nails

Normal

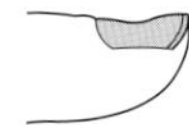

Koilonychia

can occur in *cirrhosis*

  - koilonychia—misshapen, concave nails (Figure 2.2)

can occur in *iron-deficiency anaemia*

  - clubbing—loss of angle at base of nail (Figure 2.3)

Occurs in specific diseases:

- heart: *infectious endocarditis, cyanotic congenital heart disease*

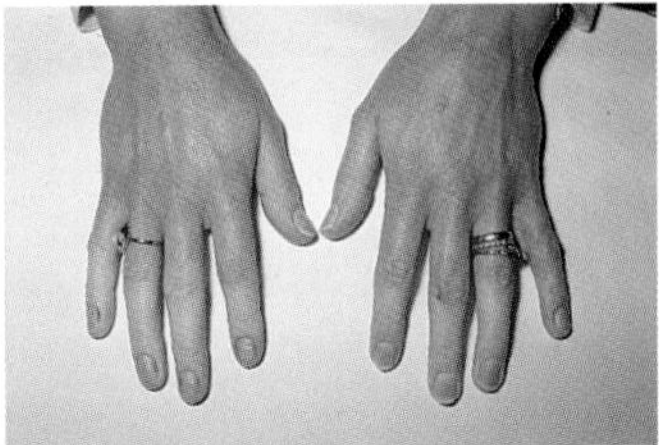

Figure 2.1 Raynaud's syndrome—white/blue fingers induced by cold.

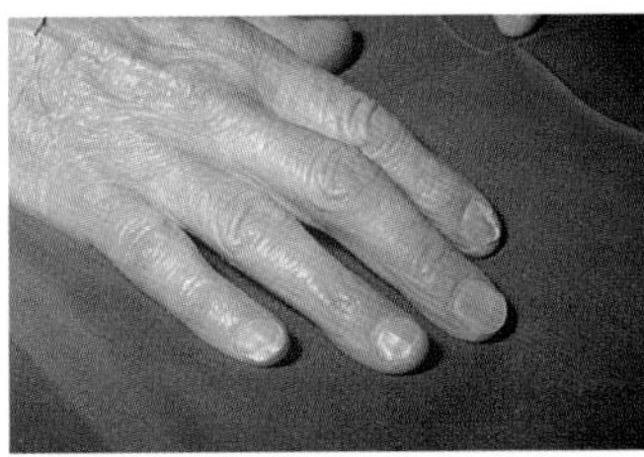

Figure 2.2 Koilonychia from iron deficiency—spoon-shaped nails.

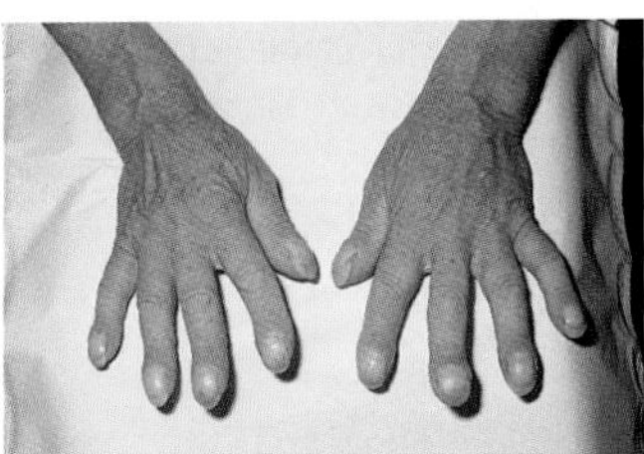

Figure 2.3 Finger clubbing—gross with carcinoma of bronchus.

- lungs: *carcinoma of the bronchus* (*chronic infection*; *abscess*; *bronchiectasis*, e.g. *cystic fibrosis*; *empyema*); *fibrosing alveolitis* (not chronic bronchitis)
- liver: *cirrhosis*
- *Crohn's disease*
- *congenital*.

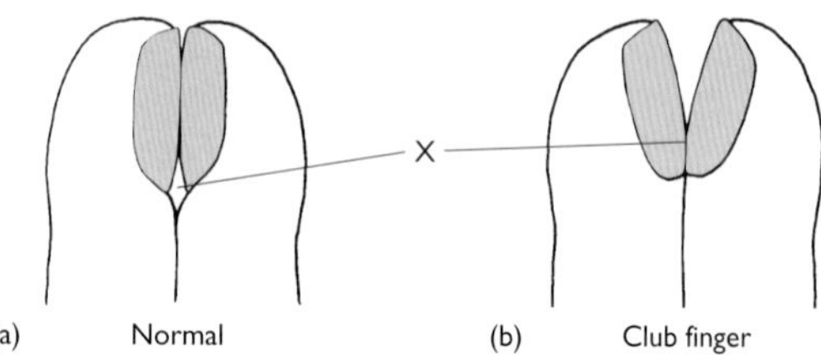

- splinter haemorrhages—occur in *infectious endocarditis* but are more common in people doing manual work (Figure 2.4)
- pitting—*psoriasis*
- onycholysis—separation of nail from nail bed—*psoriasis, thyrotoxicosis*
- paronychia—pustule in lateral nail fold.

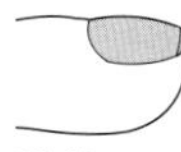

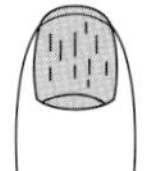

- **Palms:**
  - erythema—can be normal, also occurs with *chronic liver disease, pregnancy*
  - Dupuytren's contracture (Figure 2.5)—tethering of skin in palm to flexor tendon of fourth finger, may be related to *cirrhosis* or familial.
- **Joints:**
  - symmetrical swellings occur in *rheumatoid arthritis* (Figure 2.6)

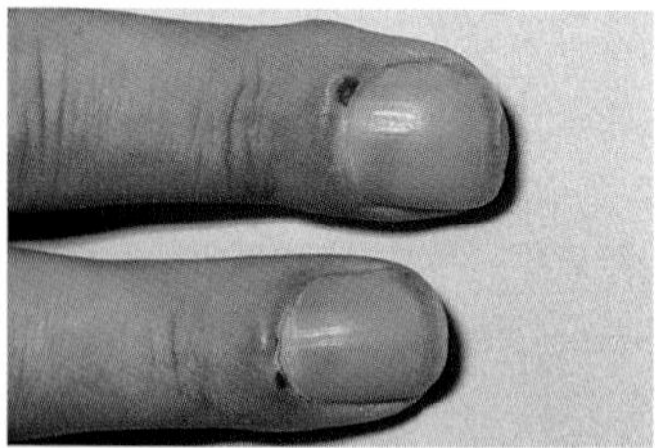

Figure 2.4 Nail-fold infarcts from polyarteritis—small black areas, often associated with splinter haemorrhages in nails.

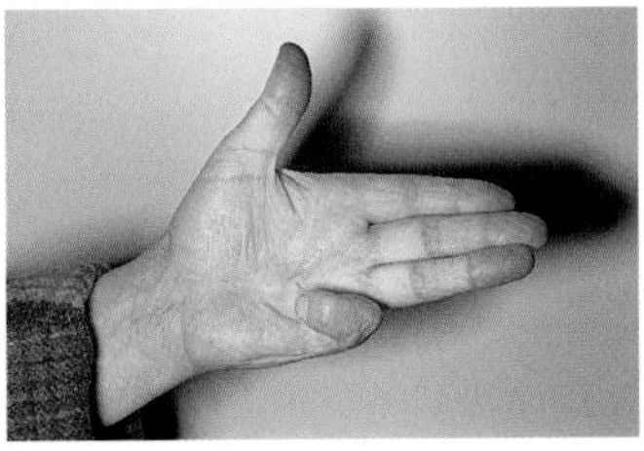

Figure 2.5 Dupuytren's contraction—thickened palmar skin attached to the tendons.

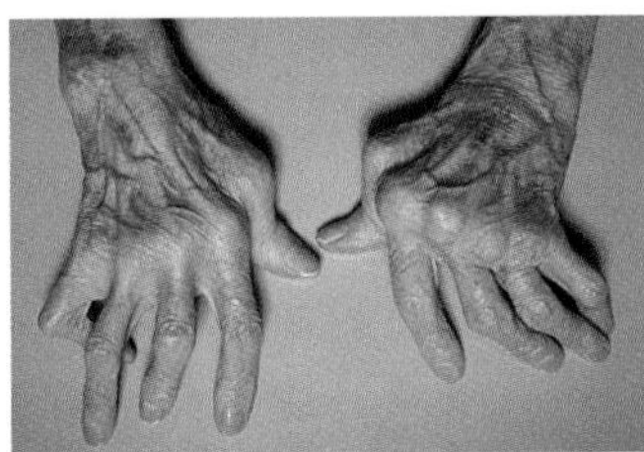

Figure 2.6 Rheumatoid arthritis—symmetrically enlarged metacarpophalangeal and interphalangeal joints, with secondary wasting of interossei muscles and subluxation of fingers from snapped dorsal tendons.

- asymmetrical swellings occur in *gout* (Figure 2.7) and *osteoarthritis*.

Skin

Inspection of skin

- distribution of any lesions from end of bed
- examine close up with palpation of skin
- remember mucous membranes, hair and nails.

- **Colour:**
  - pigmented apart from racial pigmentation or suntan—examine buccal mucosa
  - if appears jaundiced—examine sclerae
  - if pale—examine conjunctivae for anaemia.
- **Skin texture:**
  - ? normal for age—becomes thinner from age 50
  - thin, e.g. *Cushing's syndrome, hypothyroid, hypopituitary, malnutrition, liver or renal failure*

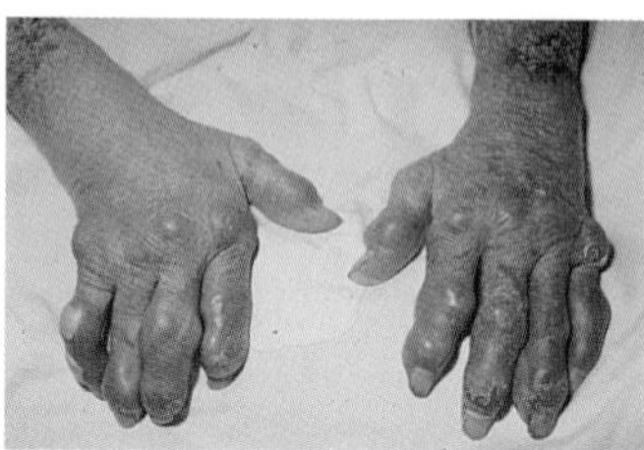

Figure 2.7 Gout—asymmetrical swelling of joints with subcutaneous 'tophi' of uric acid deposits.

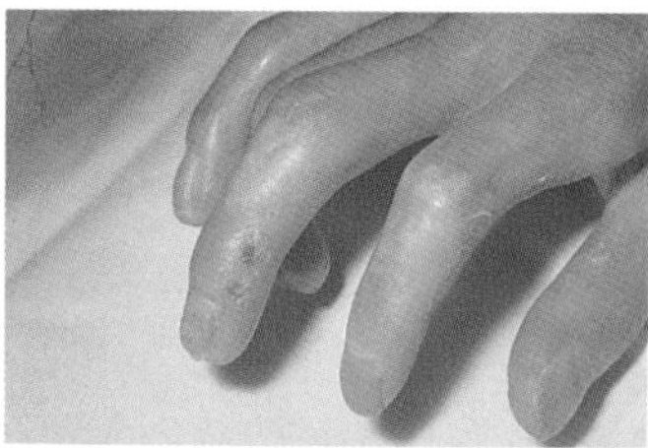

Figure 2.8 Scleroderma—thick shiny skin and limiting joint movements with ulcers from subcutaneous calcification.

  - thick, e.g. *acromegaly, androgen excess*
  - dry, e.g. *hypothyroid*
  - tethered, e.g. *scleroderma* of fingers, attached to underlying breast tumour (Figure 2.8).
- **Rash:**
  - what is it like? Describe precisely.

Inspection of lesions

- distribution of lesions:
  - symmetrical or asymmetrical
  - peripheral or mainly on trunk
  - maximal on light-exposed sites
  - pattern of contact with known agents, e.g. shoes, gloves, cosmetics
- number and size of lesions
- look at an early lesion
- discrete or confluent

- pattern of lesions, e.g. linear, annular, serpiginous (like a snake), reticular (like a net)
- is edge well-demarcated?
- colour
- surface, e.g. scaly, shiny

Palpation of lesions

- flat, impalpable—*macular*
- raised
  - *papular:* in skin, localised
  - *plaque:* larger, e.g. >0.5 cm
  - *nodules:* deeper in dermis, persisting more than 3 days
  - *wheal:* oedema fluid, transient, less than 3 days
  - *vesicles:* contain fluid (Figure 2.9)
  - *bullae:* large vesicles, e.g. >0.5 cm
  - *pustular*
- deep in dermis—*nodules*
- temperature
- tender?
- blanches on pressure—most erythematous lesions, e.g. *drug rash*, *telangiectasia*, dilated capillaries (Figure 2.10)
- does not blanch on pressure

Purpura or *petechiae* are small discrete microhaemorrhages approximately 1 mm across, red, non-tender macules.

If palpable, suggests *vasculitis* (Figure 2.11).

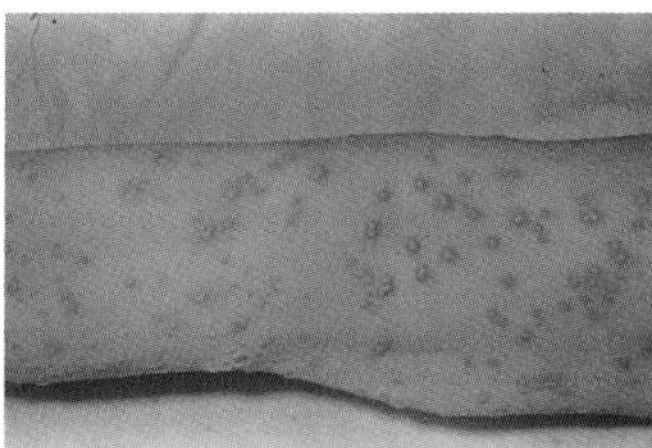

Figure 2.9 Chicken pox—peripheral circumscribed, erythematous papules with central blister.

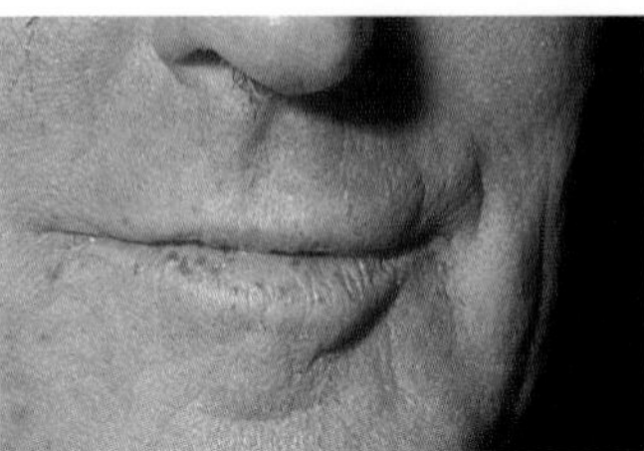

Figure 2.10 Osler–Weber–Rendu syndrome—telangiectasia on the lip in a patient with haematemasis.

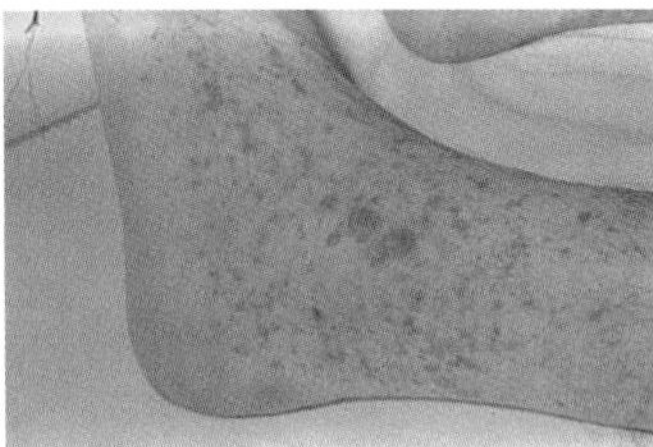

Figure 2.11 Henoch–Schönlein syndrome—macular/papular rash including petechiae that do not blanche on pressure.

Senile purpura local haemorrhages are from minor traumas in thin skin of hands or forearms. Flat purple/brown lesions.

- hard
- sclerosis, e.g. *scleroderma* of fingers (Figure 2.8)
- infiltration, e.g. *lymphoma* or *cancer*
- scars

Enquire about the time course of any lesion

- 'How long has it been there?'
- 'Is it fixed in size and position? Does it come and go?'
- 'Is it itchy, sore, tender or anaesthetic?'

Knowledge of the differential diagnosis will indicate other questions:

- dermatitis of hand—contact with chemicals or plants, wear and tear

- ulcer of toe—*arterial disease, diabetes mellitus, neuropathy*
- pigmentation and ulcer of lower medial leg—*varicose veins.*

Common diseases

Acne	Pilar-sebaceous follicular inflammation—papules and pustules on face and upper trunk, blackheads (*comedones*), cysts.
Basal cell carcinoma (rodent ulcer) (Figure 2.12)	Shiny papule with rolled border and capillaries on surface. Can have a depressed centre or ulcerate.
Bullae	Blisters due to burns, infection of the skin, allergy or, rarely, autoimmune diseases affecting adhesion within epidermis (*pemphigus*) or at the epidermal–dermal junction (*pemphigoid*).
Café-au-lait patches	Permanent discrete brown macules of varying size and shape. If large and numerous, suggests neurofibromatosis.
Drug eruptions (Figure 2.13)	Usually macular, symmetrical distribution. Can be urticaria, eczematous and various forms, including erythema multiforme or erythema nodosum (see below).

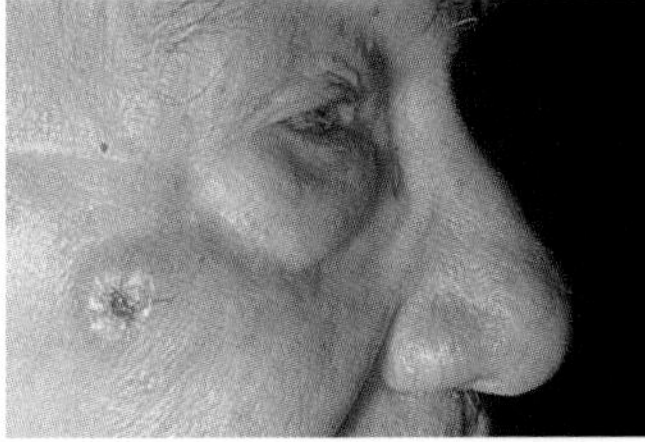

Figure 2.12 Rodent ulcer—raised, shiny papule with telangiectasia on the surface with a central ulcer.

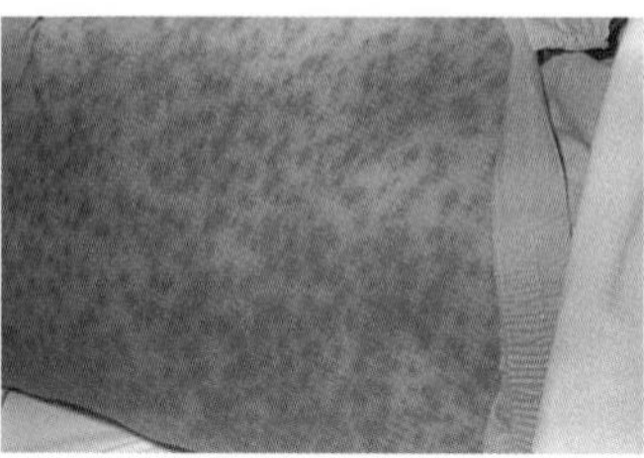

Figure 2.13 Ampicillin rash—patchy red macules that blanche on pressure.

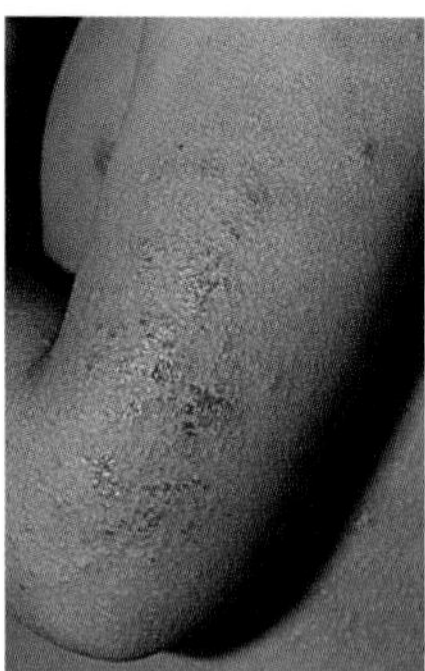

Figure 2.14 Eczema on upper arm—diffuse erythema and scratch marks, with small blisters and fine scales that cannot be seen on this photo.

Eczema (Figure 2.14)	*Atopic dermatitis:* dry skin, red, plaques, commonly on the face, antecubital and popliteal fossae, with fine scales, vesicles and scratch marks secondary to *pruritus* (itching). Often associated with *asthma* and *hayfever*. Family history of atopy. *Contact dermatitis:* may be irritant or allergic. Red, scaly plaques with vesicles in acute stages.
Erythema multiforme	Symmetrical, widespread inflammatory 0.5–1 cm macules/

	papules, often with central blister. Can be confluent. Usually on hands and feet: *drug reactions* *viral infections* *no apparent cause* *Stevens–Johnson syndrome*—with mucosal desquamation involving genitalia, mouth and conjunctivae, with fever.
Erythema nodosum (Figure 2.15)	Tender, localised, red, diffusely raised, 2–4 cm nodules in anterior shins. Due to: *streptococcal infection*, e.g. with *rheumatic fever* *primary tuberculosis* and other infections *sarcoid* *inflammatory bowel disease* *drug reactions* *no apparent cause*.
Fungus	Red, annular, scaly area of skin. When involving the nails, they become thickened with loss of compact structure.
Herpes infection (Figure 2.16)	Clusters of vesicopustules which crust, recurs at the same site, e.g. lips, genitalia.

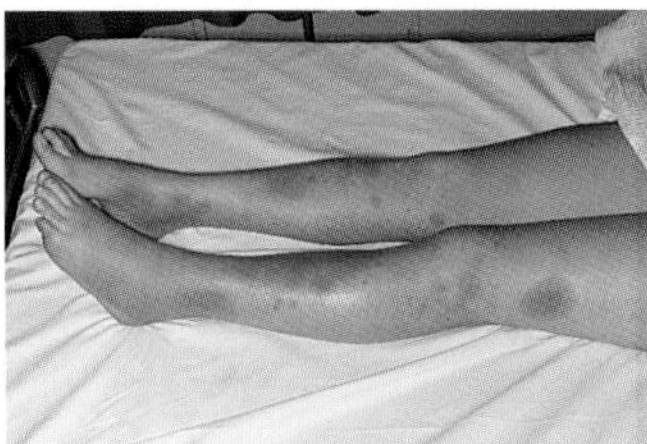

Figure 2.15 Erythema nodosum—approximately 5–10 cm across swellings in dermis of shins with red, warm surfaces.

Impetigo	Spreading pustules and yellow crusts from staphylococcal infection.
Malignant melanoma	Usually irregular pigmented, papule or plaque, superficial or thick with irregular edge, enlarging with tendency to bleed.
Psoriasis (Figure 2.17)	Symmetrical eruption: chronic, discrete, red plaques with silvery scales. Gentle scraping easily induces bleeding. Often affects scalp, elbows and knees. Nails may be pitted. Familial and precipitated by streptococcal sore throats or skin trauma.

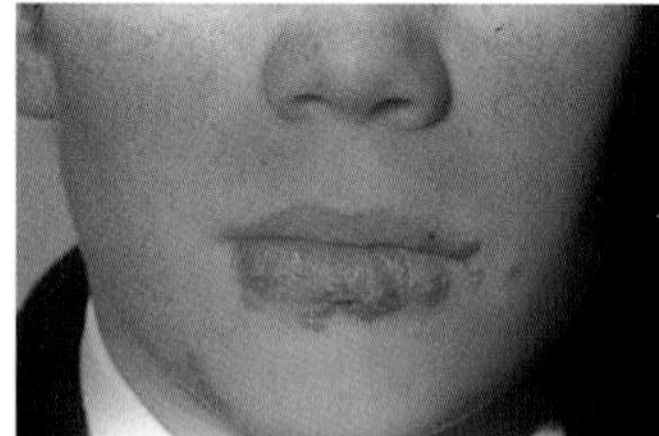

Figure 2.16 Herpes simplex on lips ('cold sores')—these can erupt with other illnesses.

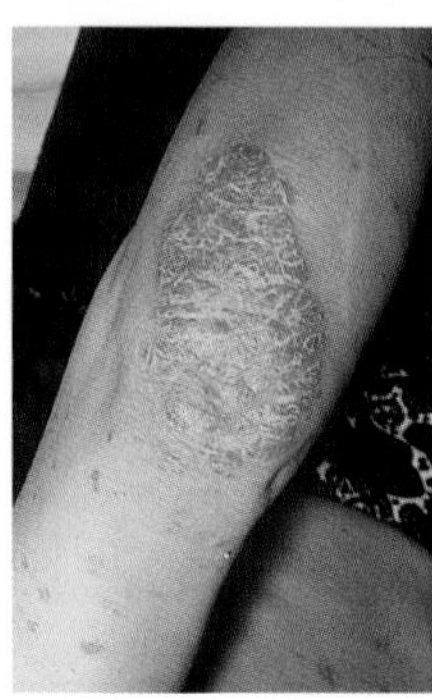

Figure 2.17 Psoriasis—circumscribed plaque with scales.

Scabies	Mite infection: itching, with 2–4 mm tunnels in epidermis, e.g. in webs of fingers, wrists, genitalia.
Squamous cell carcinoma	Warty localised thickening, may ulcerate.
Urticaria	Transient wheal with surrounding erythema. Lasts around 24 hours. Usually allergic to drugs, e.g. aspirin, or physical, e.g. dermographism, cold.
Vitiligo	Permanent demarcated, depigmented white patches due to autoimmune disease.

Mouth

- **Look at the tongue:**
  - cyanosed, moist or dry.

Cyanosis is a reduction in the oxygenation of the blood, with more than 5 g/dl deoxygenated haemoglobin.

Central cyanosis (blue tongue) denotes a right-to-left shunt (unsaturated blood appearing in systemic circulation):

- congenital heart disease, e.g. *Fallot's tetralogy* (Figure 2.18)
- lung disease, e.g. *obstructive airways disease*.

Peripheral cyanosis (blue fingers, pink tongue) denotes inadequate peripheral circulation.

A dry tongue can mean salt and water deficiency (often called 'dehydration') but also occurs with mouth-breathing.

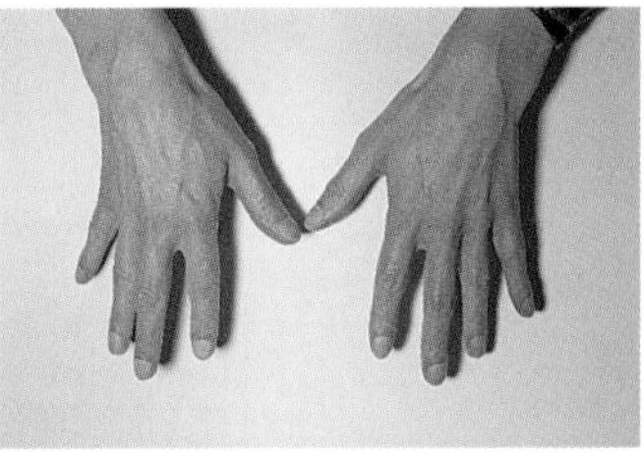

Figure 2.18 Congenital cyanotic heart disease—dusky, cyanotic hands with mild clubbing.

- **Look at the teeth:**
  - caries (exposed dentine), poor dental hygiene, false.
- **Look at the gums:**
  - bleeding, swollen.
- **Look at: redness, exudate**
  - tonsils
  - pharynx: swelling, redness, ulceration.
- **Smell patient's breath:**
  - ketosis
  - alcohol
  - foetor

    constipation, appendicitis

    musty in liver failure.

Ketosis is a sweet-smelling breath occurring with *starvation* or *severe diabetes*.

Hepatic foetor is a musty smell in *liver failure*.

Eyes

- **Look at the eyes:**
  - *sclera*, icterus

The most obvious demonstration of *jaundice* is the yellow sclera (Figure 2.19).

- *lower lid conjunctiva*, anaemia

Anaemia. If the lower lid is everted, the colour of the mucous membrane can be seen. If these are pale, the haemoglobin is usually less than 9 g/dl.

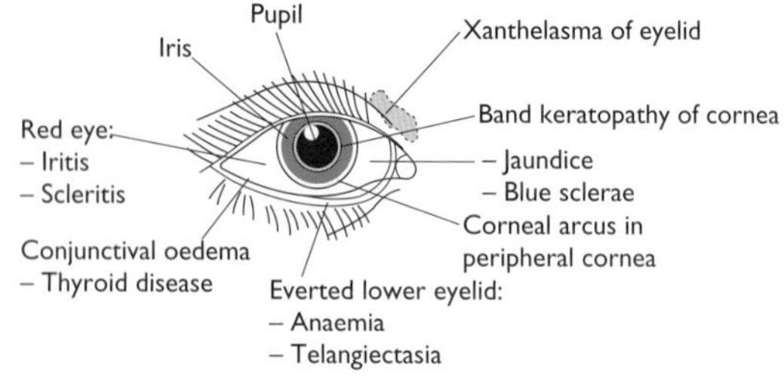

- eyelids: white/yellow deposit, *xanthelasma*

- puffy eyelids

general oedema, e.g. *nephrotic syndrome*
thyroid eye disease, hyper or hypo
myxoedema

- red eye
  - *iritis*
  - *conjunctivitis*
  - *scleritis* or *episcleritis*
  - *acute glaucoma*

- white line around cornea, *arcus senilis*

common and of little significance in the elderly
suggests *hyperlipidaemia* in younger patients (Figure 2.20)

- white-band keratopathy-hypercalcaemia

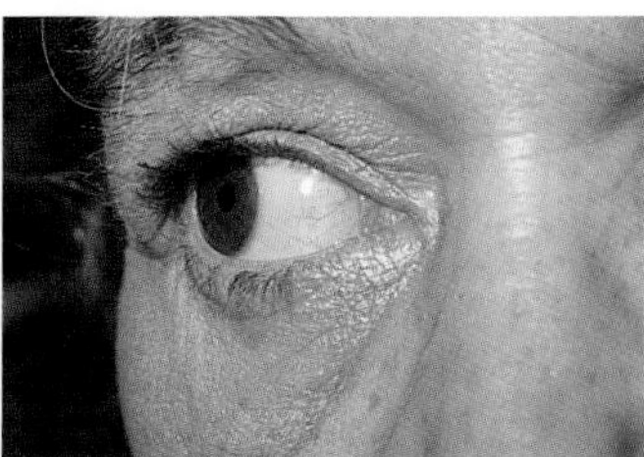

Figure 2.19 Jaundice—yellow sclerae.

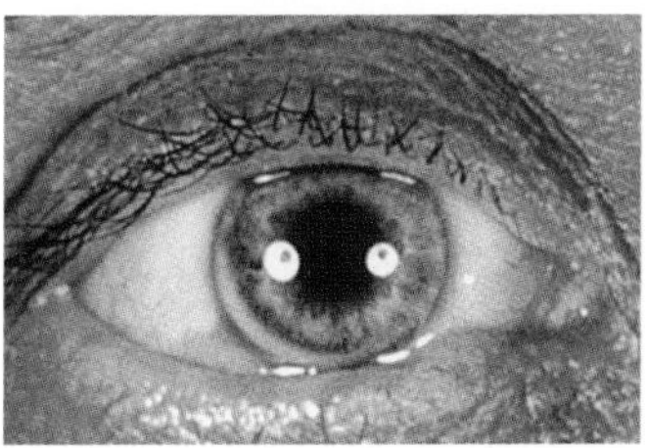

Figure 2.20 Corneal arcus—same age relationship as xanthelasma.

- *sarcoid*
- *parathyroid tumour* or *hyperplasia*
- *lung oat-cell tumour*
- *bone secondaries*
- *vitamin D excess intake*
- *hypercalcaemia* may give a horizontal band across exposed medial and lateral parts of cornea.

Examine the fundi

This is often done as part of the neurological system, when examining the cranial nerves. It is placed here as features cover general medicine.

- **Use ophthalmoscope**
  - The patient should be sitting. Start examination at 1 m from the patient, identify red reflex and approach the patient at an angle of 15° to the patient. Approach on the same horizontal plane as patient's equator of their eye. This will bring the observer straight to the optic disc. After observing the disc examine the peripheral retina fully by following the blood vessels to and back from the four main quadrants.
  - Use your right eye for patient's right eye, left eye for patient's left eye.
- **Look at optic disc**
  - normally pink rim with white 'cup' below surface of disc:

optic atrophy

- disc pale, rim no longer pink:
  - *multiple sclerosis*
  - *after optic neuritis*
  - *optic nerve compression*, e.g. *tumour*
- papilloedema
  - disc pink, indistinct margin
  - cup disappears
  - dilated retinal veins:

increased cerebral pressure, e.g. *tumour*

accelerated hypertension
optic neuritis, acute stage

- glaucoma—enlarged cup, diminished rim
- new vessels—new fronds of vessels coming forward from disc:

ischaemic diabetic retinopathy.

- **Look at arteries (Figure 2.21)**
  - arteries narrowed in hypertension, with increased light reflex along top of vessel

Hypertension grading:

1 narrow arteries
2 'nipping' (narrowing of veins by arteries)
3 flame-shaped haemorrhages and cotton-wool spots
4 papilloedema.

(a) 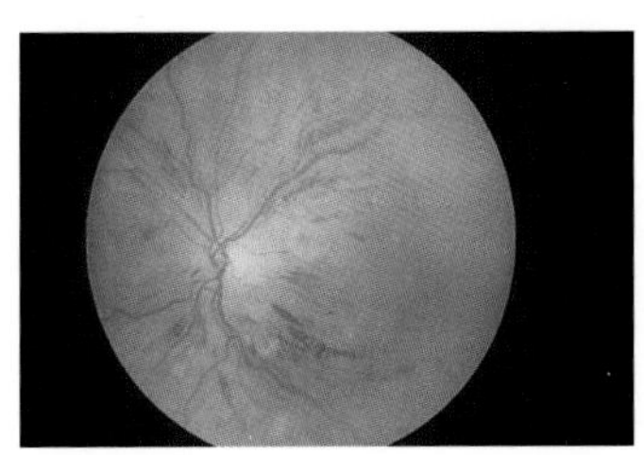 (reversed)

Hypertensive retinopathy

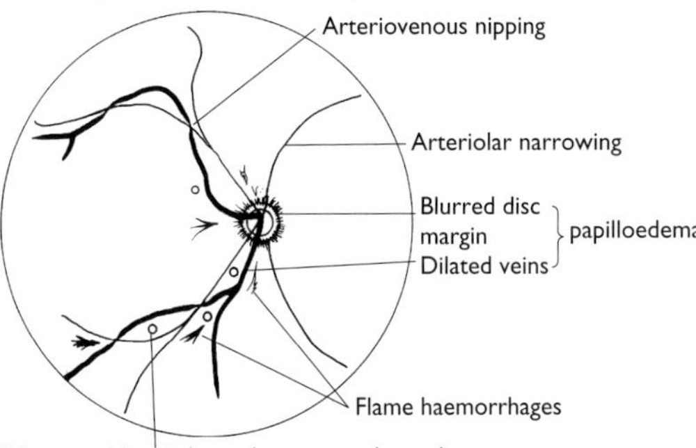

(b)

Figure 2.21 Hypertensive retinopathy—narrow arteries, flame haemorrhages and an early papilloedema with an indistinct disc margin.

    - occlusion artery—pale retina
    - occlusion vein—haemorrhages.
- **Look at retina (Figure 2.22)**
    - hard exudates (shiny, yellow circumscribed patches of lipid):

diabetes

- cotton-wool spots (soft, fluffy white patches)
    - microinfarcts causing local swelling of nerve fibres:

diabetes
hypertension
vasculitis
human immunodeficiency virus (HIV)

(a)
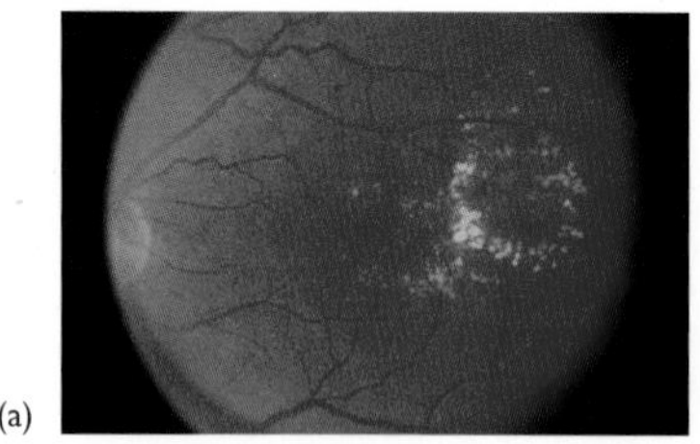
(reversed)

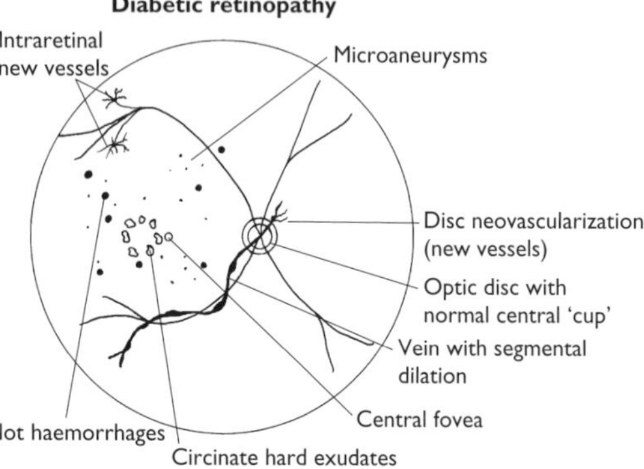

(b)

Figure 2.22 Diabetic retinopathy—hard exudates in a ring (circinate).

- small, red dots
    - microaneurysms—retinal capillary expansion adjacent to capillary closure:

diabetes

- haemorrhages
    - round 'blots': haemorrhages deep in retina
    - larger than microaneurysms:

diabetes

- flame-shaped: superficial haemorrhages along nerve fibres:

hypertension
gross anaemia
hyperviscosity
bleeding tendency

- Roth's spots (white-centred haemorrhages)

microembolic disorder
subacute bacterial endocarditis

- pigmentation
    - widespread:

retinitis pigmentosa

- localised:

choroiditis (clumping of pigment into patches)
drug toxicity, e.g. chloroquine

- tigroid or tabby fundus: normal variant in choroid beneath retina
- peripheral new vessels:

ischaemic diabetic retinopathy
retinal vein occlusion

- medullated nerve fibres—normal variant, areas of white nerves radiating from optic disc.

Examine for palpable lymph nodes

- In the neck:
    - above clavicle (posterior triangle, supraclavicular)

- medial to sternomastoid area (anterior triangle, anterior cervical chain)
- submandibular (can palpate submandibular gland)
- submental

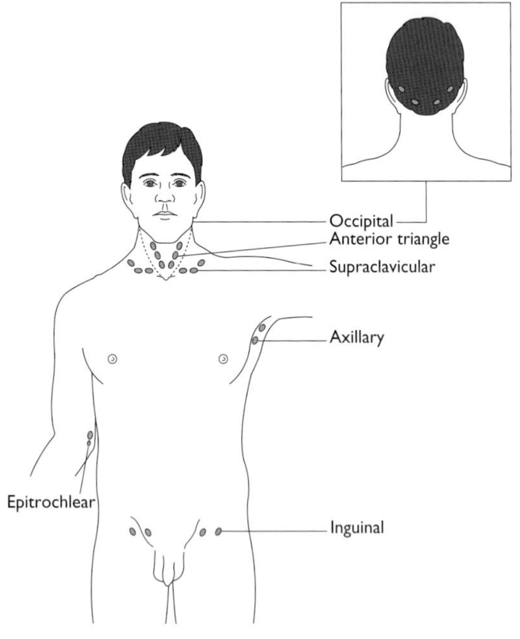

- pre-auricular
- post-auricular
- occipital.

These glands are best felt by sitting the patient up and examining from behind. A left supraclavicular node can occur from the spread of a gastrointestinal malignancy (Virchow's node).

- In the axillae:
  - abduct arm, insert your hand along lateral side of axilla and adduct arm, thus placing your fingertips in the apex of the axilla. Palpate gently, feel the

medial, lateral, anterior, posterior and apical groups of nodes.

- In the epitrochlear region:
  - medial to and above elbow.
- In the groins:
  - over inguinal ligament and femoral triangle (medial to femoral pulse).
- In the abdomen:
  - usually very difficult to feel, you may feel an enlarged spleen

- Axillae often have soft, fleshy lymph nodes.
- Groins often have small, shotty nodes.
- Generalised large, rubbery nodes suggest *lymphoma*.
- Localised hard nodes suggest *cancer*.
- Tender nodes suggest *infection*.

If many nodes are palpable—examine spleen and look for anaemia. *Lymphoma* or *leukaemia*?

Lumps

- If there is an unusual lump, **inspect first and palpate later**:
  - **site**
  - **size** (measure in centimetres)
  - **shape**
  - **colour**
  - **surface, edge**
  - **surroundings**
  - **fixed or mobile** (relation to underlying structures)
  - **consistency**, e.g. cystic or solid, soft or hard, fluctuance
  - **tender**
  - **pulsatile**
  - **auscultation** (for bruit or bowel sounds)
  - **transillumination**.

A *cancer* is usually hard, non-tender, irregular, fixed to neighbouring tissues, and possibly ulcerating skin.
A *cyst* may have:

- **fluctuance**: pressure across cyst will cause it to bulge in another plane
- **transillumination**: a light can be seen through it (usually only if room is darkened).

- Look at neighbouring lymph nodes. May find:
  - spread from cancer
  - inflamed lymph nodes from infection.

Ulcers

- This is an area of loss of the normal epithelial/ endothelial covering. When inspecting the skin, make specific note of the following:
  - **site**
  - **size** (measure in centimetres)
  - **shape**
  - **depth**
  - **edge** (rolled or discrete)
  - **base** (healing with pink granulation or sloughy)
  - **underlying tissue involvement** (e.g. tendons, muscle, bone)
  - **associated venous disease** (e.g. varicose veins, oedema, lipodermatosclerosis)
  - **palpate for pulses** (to exclude arterial insufficiency as a cause)
  - **history of trauma**.

Breasts

Unless impossible, arrange a female chaperone, particularly when the patient is a young adult, shy or nervous.

Routine examination

- Examine the female breasts **when you examine the precordium**.
- **Inspect for asymmetry**, obvious lumps, inverted nipples, skin changes.
- **Palpate each quadrant of both breasts** with the flat of the hand (fingers together, nearly extended with

gentle pressure exerted from metacarpophalangeal joints, avoiding pressure on the nipple).
- If there are any possible lumps, proceed to a more complete examination.

Full breast examination

When patient has a symptom or a lump has been found:
- **Inspect**
  - **sitting up and ask the patient to raise hands**
  - **inspect for asymmetry** or obvious lumps
    - differing size or shape of breasts
    - nipples—symmetry
    - rashes, redness (abscess)

  Breast cancer is suggested by:
  - asymmetry
  - skin tethering
  - *peau d'orange* (oedema of skin)
  - nipple deviated or inverted.

- **Palpate**
  - patient lying flat, one pillow
  - **examine each breast with flat of hand, each quadrant in turn and behind the nipple**
  - examine bimanually if large
  - examine any lump as described above
    - is lump attached to skin or muscles?
    - examine lymph nodes (axilla and supraclavicular)
    - feel liver.

Thyroid

- **Inspect**: then ask the patient to swallow, having given them a glass of water. Is there a lump? Does it move upwards on swallowing?
- **Palpate bimanually**: stand behind the patient and palpate with fingers of both hands. Is the thyroid of normal size, shape and texture?
- If a lump is felt:
  - is thyroid multinodular?
  - does lump feel cystic?

The thyroid is normally soft. If there is a goitre (swelling of thyroid), assess if the swelling is:

- localised, e.g. *thyroid cyst, adenoma* or *carcinoma*
- generalised, e.g. *autoimmune thyroiditis, thyrotoxicosis*
- multinodular.

A swelling does not mean the gland is under- or overactive. In many cases the patient may be euthyroid. The thyroid becomes slightly enlarged in pregnancy.

- **Ask patient to swallow**—does thyroid rise normally?
- Is thyroid fixed?
- **Can you get below the lump?** If not, percuss over upper sternum for retrosternal extension.
- **Are there cervical lymph nodes?**
- **If possibility of patient being thyrotoxic (Figure 2.23 and 2.24), look for:**
  - warm hands
  - perspiration
  - tremor
  - tachycardia, sinus rhythm or atrial fibrillation
  - wide, palpable fissure or lid lag
  - thyroid bruit (on auscultation).

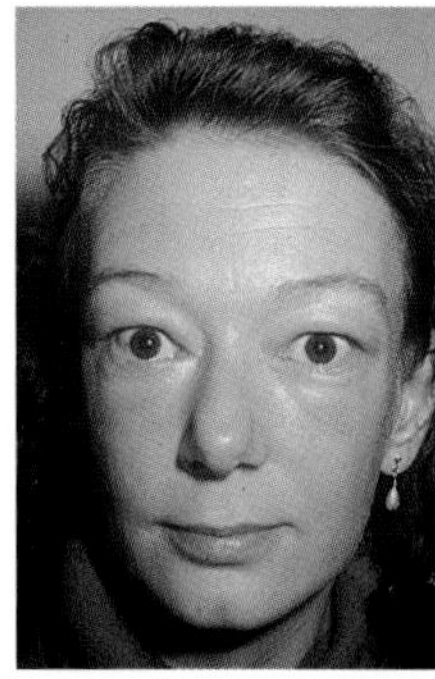

Figure 2.23 Thyrotoxicosis—wide palpebral fissures in a tense person.

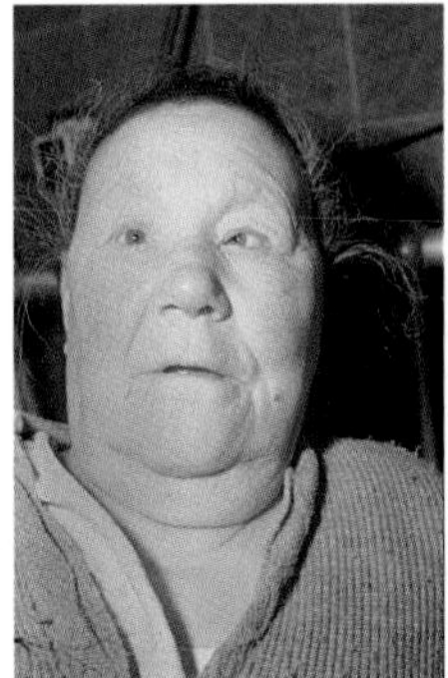

Figure 2.24 Myxoedema—puffy face, thin dry hair and dry skin in a sluggish person.

Endocrine exophthalmos (may be associated with thyrotoxicosis):
- conjunctival oedema: *chemosis* (seen by gentle pressure on lower lid, pushing up a fold of conjunctiva when oedema is present)
- proptosis: eye pushed forwards (look from above down on eyes)
- deficient upward gaze and convergence
- diplopia
- papilloedema.

- If possibility of patient being *hypothyroid*, look for:
  - dry hair and skin
  - xanthelasma
  - puffy face
  - croaky voice
  - delayed relaxation of supinator or ankle jerks.

Other endocrine diseases

Acromegaly (Figure 2.25)

- enlarged soft tissue of hands, feet, face
- coarse features, thick, greasy skin, large tongue (and other organs, e.g. thyroid)
- bitemporal hemianopia (from tumour pressing on optic chiasma) (Figure 2.25)

Hypopituitary

- no skin pigmentation
- thin skin

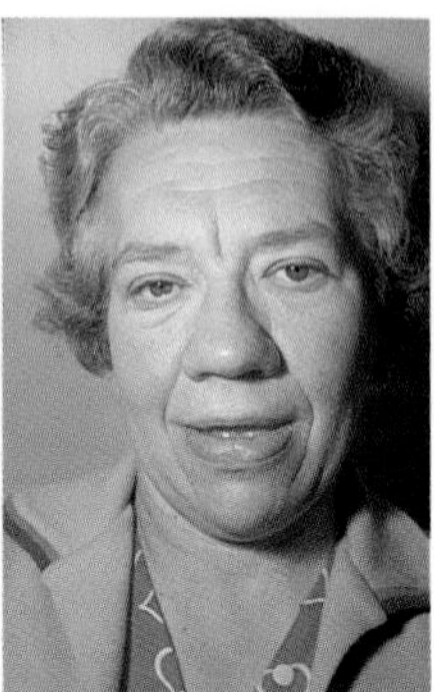

Figure 2.25 Acromegaly—coarse features with thick lips, enlarged nose and thickened skin.

- decreased secondary sexual hair or delayed puberty
- short stature (and on X-ray, delayed fusion of epiphyses)
- bitemporal hemianopia if pituitary tumour

Addison's disease

- increased skin pigmentation, including non-exposed areas, e.g. buccal pigmentation
- postural hypotension
- if female, decreased body hair

Cushing's syndrome (Figure 2.26)

- truncal obesity, round, red face with hirsutism
- thin skin and bruising, pink striae, hypertension
- proximal muscle weakness

Diabetes

Diabetic complications include:

- skin lesions

Necrobiosis lipoidica—ischaemia in skin, usually on shins, leading to fatty replacement of dermis, covered by thin skin (Figure 2.27).

- ischaemic legs
  - diminished foot pulses
  - skin shiny blue, white or black

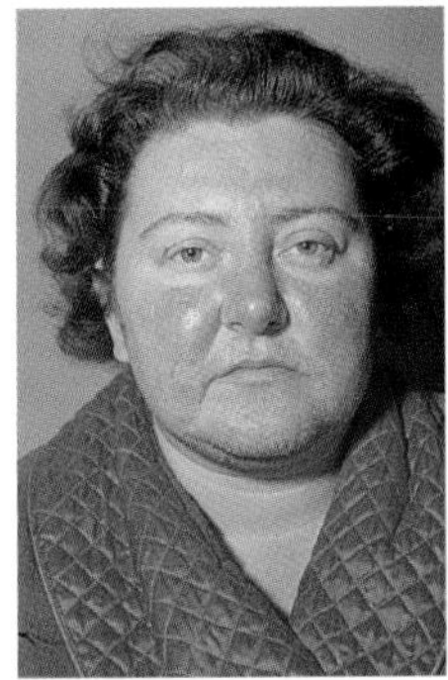

Figure 2.26 Cushing's syndrome—plethoric, round face.

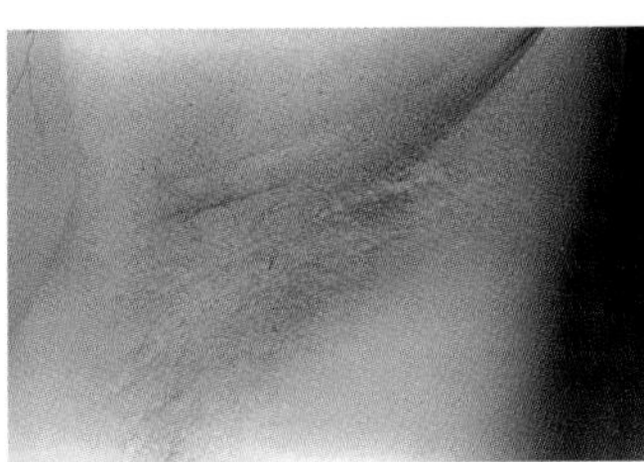

Figure 2.27 Acanthosis nigricans in the axilla—thickened epidermis from gross insulin resistance which also occurs on the neck.

    - no hairs, thick nails
    - ulcers
- peripheral neuropathy
    - absent leg reflexes
    - diminished sensation
    - thick skin over unusual pressure points from dropped arch
- autonomic neuropathy
    - dry skin
- mononeuropathy
    - lateral popliteal nerve—footdrop
    - III or VI—diplopia
    - asymmetrical muscle-wasting of the upper leg
- retinopathy (Figure 2.22).

Locomotor system

Normally one examines joints briefly when examining neighbouring systems. If a patient specifically complains of joint symptoms or an abnormal posture or joint is noted, a more detailed examination is needed. A general plan for the locomotor system is Look, Feel, Move (inspection, palpation, movements).

General habitus

- Note the following:
  - is the patient unduly tall or short? Measure height and span
  - are all limbs, spine and skull of normal size and shape?
    - normal person:

height = span
crown to pubis = pubis to heel

- long limbs:

Marfan's syndrome
eunuchoid during growth

- *collapsed vertebrae:*

span > height
pubis to heel > crown to pubis

- is the posture normal?
- curvature of the spine:

flexion: *kyphosis*
extension: *lordosis*
lateral: *scoliosis*

Flexion

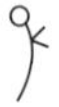

Extension

Lateral

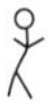

- is the gait normal?

Observing the patient walking is a vital part of examination of the locomotor system and neurological system.

Painful gait, transferring weight quickly off a painful limb, bobbing up and down—an abnormal rhythm of gait.

Painless abnormal gait may be from:
short leg (bobs up and down with equal-length steps)

stiff joint (lifts pelvis to prevent foot dragging on ground)
weak ankle (high stepping gait to avoid toes catching on ground)
weak knee (locks knee straight before putting foot on the ground)
weak hip (sways sideways using trunk muscles to lift pelvis and to swing leg through)
uncoordinated gait (arms are swung as counterbalances)
hysterical or malingering causes.

Look for abnormal wear on shoes.

Inspection

- Inspect the joints before you touch them.
- Look at:
  - skin
    redness—inflammation
    scars—old injury, surgery
    bruising—recent injury
  - soft tissues
    muscle wasting—old injury, neurological disease
    swelling—injury/inflammation
  - bones
    deformity—compare with other side

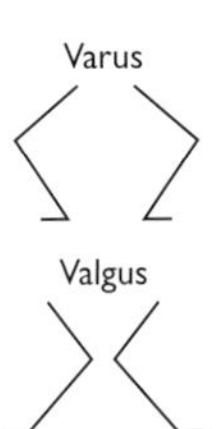

varus: bent in to midline
valgus: bent out from midline.

- Assess whether an isolated joint is affected, or if there is polyarthritis.
- If there is polyarthritis, note if it is symmetrical or asymmetrical.
- Compare any abnormal findings with the other side, in fact usually examine the 'normal' side first as a comparison.

  - *Arthritis*—swollen, hot, tender, painful joint.
  - *Arthropathy*—swollen but not hot and tender.
  - *Arthralgia*—painful, e.g. on movement, without being swollen.

  Swelling may also be due to an effusion, thickening of the periarticular tissues, enlargement of the ends of bones (e.g.

pulmonary osteopathy) or complete disorganisation of the joint without pain (*Charcot's joint*).

Palpation

- Before you touch any joint ask the patient to tell you if it is painful.
- Feel for:
  - warmth
  - tenderness
    - watch patient's face for signs of discomfort
    - locate signs of tenderness—soft tissue or bone
  - swelling or displacement
  - fluctuation (effusion).

An inflamed joint is usually generally tender. Localised tenderness may be mechanical in origin, e.g. ligament tear. Joint effusion may occur with an arthritis or local injury.

Movement

Test the range of movement of the joint both actively and passively. This must be done **gently**.

- **Active**—how far can the patient move the joint through its range?

Do not seize limb and move it until patient complains.

- **Passive**—if range is limited, can you further increase the range of movement?

  - Abduction: movement from central axis
  - Adduction: movement to central axis
  - Flexion
  - Extension
  - Internal rotation (hip and shoulder)
  - External rotation (hip and shoulder)
  - Eversion (ankle)
  - Inversion (ankle)

  - Is the passive range of movement similar to the active range?

Limitation of the range of movement of a joint may be due to pain, muscle spasms, contracture, inflammation or thickening of the capsules or periarticular structures, effusions into the joint space, bony or cartilaginous outgrowths or painful conditions not connected with the joint.

- **Resisted movement**—ask the patient to bend the joint while you resist movement. How much force can be developed?
- **Hold your hand round the joint** while it is moving. A grating or creaking sensation (*crepitus*) may be felt.

Crepitus is usually associated with *osteoarthritis*.

Summary of signs of common illnesses

- *Osteoarthritis*
  - 'wear and tear' of a specific joint—usually large joints
  - common in elderly or after trauma to joint
  - often involves joints of the lower limbs and is asymmetrical
  - often in the lumbar or cervical spine
  - aches after use, with deep, boring pain at night
  - Heberden's nodes—osteophytes on terminal interphalangeal joints

- *Rheumatoid arthritis*

Characteristically:
  - a polyarthritis
  - symmetrical, inflamed if active
  - involves proximal interphalangeal and metacarpophalangeal joints of hands with ulnar deviation of fingers
  - involves any large joint
  - muscle wasting from disuse atrophy
  - rheumatoid nodules on extensor surface of elbows
  - may include other signs, e.g. with splenomegaly it is *Felty's syndrome*

- *Gout*

Characteristically:
  - asymmetrical

- inflamed first metatarsophalangeal joint (big toe)—involves any joint in hand, often with tophus—hard round lump of urate by joint
  - tophi on ears

- *Psoriasis (Figure 2.17)*
  - particularly involves terminal interphalangeal joints, hips and knees
  - often with pitted nails of psoriasis as well as skin lesions

- *Ankylosing spondylitis*
  - painful, stiff spine
  - later fixed in flexed position
  - hips and other joints can be involved

System-oriented examination

On a ward round in outpatients, or 'short cases' in examinations, it is common to be asked to examine a single system. It is important to have set examination schedules in your mind, so you do not miss any salient features. You may choose a different order from those suggested if it helps you. Learn the major features by rote.

At the end of each examination chapter is such a list.

'Examine the face'

- observe skin: *rodent ulcer*
- upper face: *Paget's disease, balding, myopathy, Bell's palsy*
- eyes: *anaemia, jaundice, thyrotoxicosis, myxoedema, xanthelasma, ptosis, eye palsies, Horner's syndrome*
- lower face: *steroid therapy, acromegaly, Parkinson's disease, hemiparesis, parotid tumour, thyroid enlargement*

'Examine the eyes'

- observe: *jaundice, anaemia, arcus, ptosis, Horner's syndrome*

- examine:
  - check if patient is blind—beware of glass eye
  - movements of the eyes
    - amblyopia or palsy
    - diplopia, nystagmus/false image
  - visual acuity
  - visual fields
  - pupils: light and accommodation reflexes
  - fundi: disc, arteries and veins, retina, particularly fovea

'Examine the neck'

- inspect from front and side
  - thyroid (ask patient to swallow)
  - lymph nodes
  - raised jugular venous pressure
  - lymph glands
  - other swellings
- inspect from front
  - examine neck veins
  - feel carotid arteries
  - auscultate bruits over thyroid and carotid arteries
  - check trachea is central

'Examine the hands'

- inspect from a distance front and back
  - ask the patient to place hands on a pillow
  - ask if the hands are painful
- observe: scars, abnormal posture, lumps, features of rheumatoid disease, osteoarthritis
  - look at nails
  - check for clubbing
  - check for wasting
  - check for Dupuytren's contracture
  - check for cyanosis, anaemia, palmar erythema, nicotine staining
  - check for rheumatoid nodules at elbow if features in hands

- assess for neurological function (radial, ulnar and median nerve)
- ask about function: activities of daily living (personal and domestic)

'Examine the groin'

- inspect the lower abdomen with the patient lying down flat with one pillow
  - expose the patient from xiphisternum to the suprapubic area while maintaining dignity
  - look for obvious lumps, especially in the inguinal area
  - if there is an obvious lump ask the patient if they are able to reduce it and if so to do it
  - ask the patient to turn their head to the left and give a big cough
  - look for any cough impulse in either groin (you may do this twice)
  - ask the patient to lift their head off the bed looking for a divarication of the rectus muscle
  - feel in the inguinal region while asking the patient to cough, each side in turn
  - also look for any obvious scars on the abdomen and for an umbilical hernia
  - now ask the patient to stand up and examine the inguinal area again.
  - NEVER try to reduce an inguinal hernia with the patient standing up
  - ask to examine the scrotum for lumps at this stage and the external genitalia
  - ensure that there is a chaperone available at this stage of the examination

CHAPTER 3
Examination of the cardiovascular system

General examination

- **Examine:**
- clubbing of fingernails

  Clubbing in relation to the heart suggests *infective endocarditis* or *cyanotic heart disease*.

- cold hands with blue nails—poor perfusion, peripheral cyanosis
- tongue for central cyanosis
- conjunctivae for anaemia
- signs of dyspnoea or distress

  Assess the degree of breathlessness by checking if *dyspnoea* occurs on undressing, talking, at rest or when lying flat (*orthopnoea*).

- xanthomata:

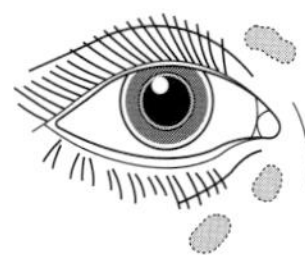
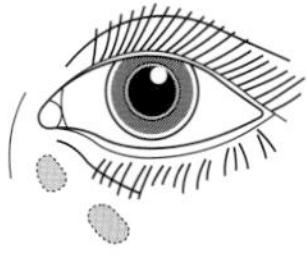

  - *xanthelasma* (common)—intracutaneous yellow cholesterol deposits occur around the eyes—normal or with *hyperlipidaemia* (Figure 3.1)
  - *xanthoma* (uncommon):
  - *hypercholesterolaemia*—tendon deposits (thickening of tendons in hands and Achilles) or tuberous

---

Clinical Skills and Examination: The Core Curriculum. By R Turner, B Angus, A Handa, C Hatton. ©2009 Blackwell Publishing, ISBN: 9781405157513.

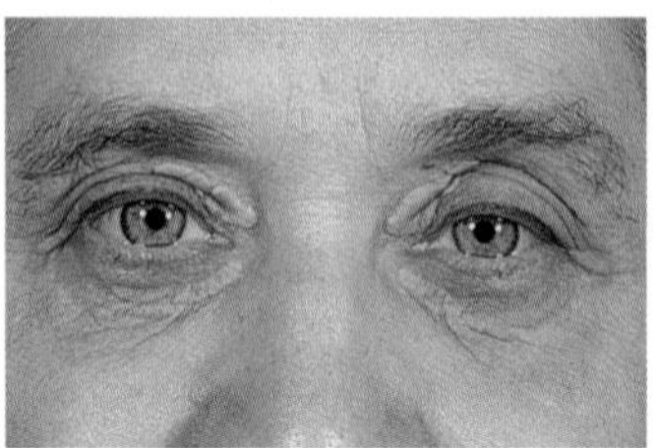

Figure 3.1 Xanthelasma–cholesterol deposits—suggests raised lipids in younger persons, but lipids are often normal in the elderly.

xanthomata yellowish patches at elbows or on eyelids (Figure 3.2)

- *hypertriglyceridaemia*—eruptive xanthoma, small yellow deposits on buttocks and extensor surfaces, each with a red halo.

Palpate the radial pulse

Feel the radial pulse just medial to the radius, with two forefingers.

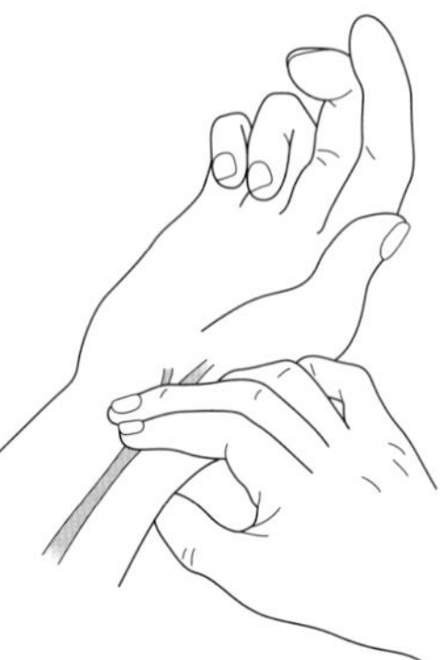

- **Pulse rate**
  Take over 15 seconds (smart alecks count for 6 seconds and multiply by 10):
  - *tachycardia* >100 beats/min
  - *bradycardia* <50 beats/min.
- **Rhythm:**
  - regular

  Normal variation on breathing: *sinus arrhythmia*.

  - regularly irregular
    - *pulsus bigeminus,* coupled extrasystoles (digoxin toxicity)
    - *Wenckebach heart block*

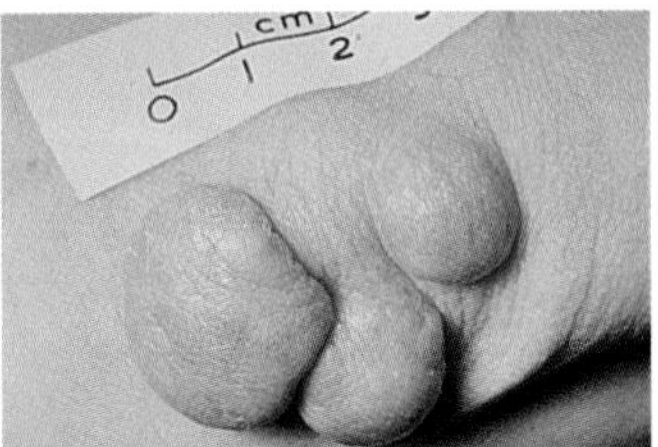

Figure 3.2 Tuberous xanthoma of elbows in homozygous familial hypercholesterolaemia—also occur in tendons and it signifies very high cholesterol levels.

- irregularly irregular
  - *multiple extrasystoles*
  - *atrial fibrillation.*

Check apical rate by auscultation for true heart rate, as small pulses are not transmitted to radial pulse.

- **Waveform of the pulse:**
  - normal (1)
  - slow rising and plateau—moderate or severe *aortic stenosis* (2)
  - collapsing pulse—pulse pressure greater than diastolic pressure, e.g. *aortic incompetence*, elderly *arteriosclerotic* patient or *gross anaemia* (3)
  - bisferiens—moderate *aortic stenosis* with severe *incompetence* (4)
  - pulsus paradoxus—pulse weaker or disappears on inspiration, e.g. *constrictive pericarditis, tamponade, status asthmaticus* (5).

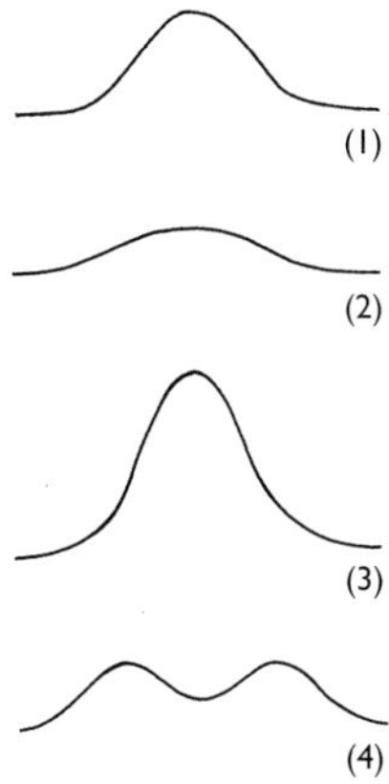

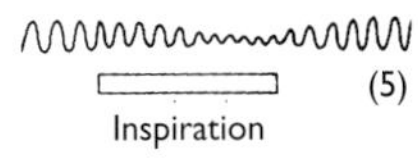

- **Volume:**
  - small volume—low cardiac output
  - large volume
    - *carbon dioxide retention*
    - *thyrotoxicosis.*
- **Stiffness of the vessel wall:**
  - in the elderly, a stiff, strongly pulsating, palpable 5–6 cm radial artery indicates *arteriosclerosis*, a hardening of the walls of the artery that is common with ageing
    - is not atheroma
    - is associated with systolic hypertension.
- **Pulsus alternans**

A difference of 20 mmHg systolic blood pressure between consecutive beats signifies poor left ventricular function. This needs to be measured with a sphygmomanometer.

Take the blood pressure

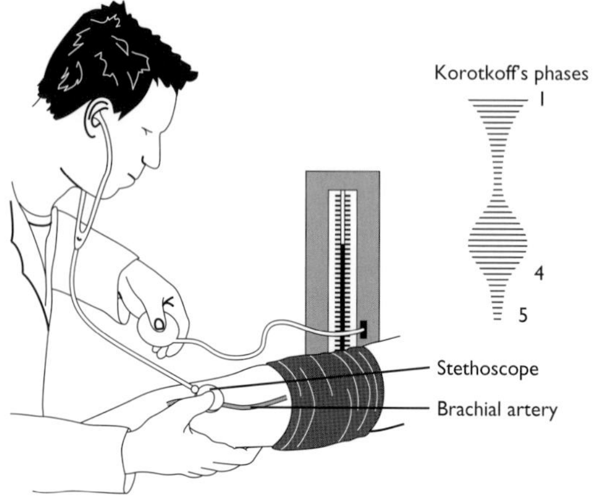

- Wrap the cuff neatly and tightly around either upper arm. The patient should be seated with the arm at the level of the heart.
- Gently inflate the cuff until the radial artery is no longer palpable.

- Using the stethoscope, listen over the brachial artery for the pulse to appear as you drop the pressure slowly (3–4 mm/s).

- Systolic blood pressure: **appearance of sounds**
  - **Korotkoff phase 1**
- Diastolic blood pressure: **disappearance of sounds**
  - **Korotkoff phase 5**

Use large cuff for fat arms (circumference >30 cm) so that inflatable cuff >1/2 arm circumference.

Beware auscultatory gap with sounds disappearing mid-systole. If sounds go to zero, use Korotkoff phase 4.

In adults, ~>1140/85 is the current guideline in non-diabetic and ~>1130/80 in diabetic patients. The patient may be nervous when first examined and the blood pressure may be falsely high. Take it again at the end of the examination.

Wide pulse pressure (e.g. 160/30 mmHg) suggests *aortic incompetence*.

Narrow pulse pressure (e.g. 95/80 mmHg) suggests *aortic stenosis*.

Difference of >20 mmHg systolic between arms suggests *arterial occlusion*, e.g. *dissecting aneurysm* or *atheroma*.

Difference of 10 mmHg is found in 25% of healthy subjects.

The variable pulse from atrial fibrillation means a precise blood pressure cannot easily be obtained.

Jugular venous pressure

- **Observe the height of the jugular venous pressure (JVP)**

Lie the patient down, resting at approximately 45° to the horizontal with their head on pillows, and shine a torch at an angle across the neck.

- **Look at the veins in the neck:**
  - internal jugular vein not directly visible: pulse diffuse, medial or deep to sternomastoid
  - external jugular vein: pulse lateral to sternomastoid. Only informative if pulsating.

- **Assess vertical height** in centimetres above the manubriosternal angle, using the pulsating external jugular vein or upper limit of internal jugular pulsation.

The **external jugular vein** is often more readily visible but may be obstructed by its tortuous course, and is less reliable than the internal jugular pulse.

The **internal jugular vein** is sometimes very difficult to see. Its pulsation may be confused with the carotid artery but it:

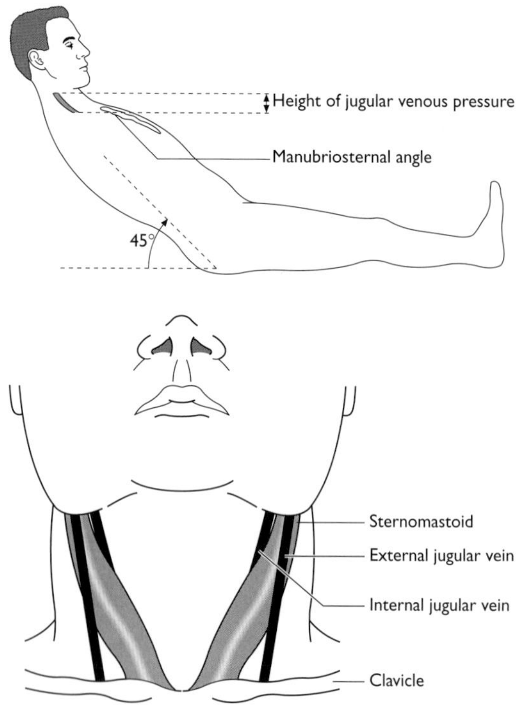

- has a complex pulsation
- moves on respiration and decreases on inspiration except in tamponade
- cannot be palpated
- can be obliterated by pressure on base of neck.

The **hepatojugular reflux** is checked by firm pressure with the flat of the right hand over the liver, while watching the JVP.

Compression on the dilated hepatic veins increases the JVP by 2 cm.

If the JVP is found to be raised above the manubriosternal angle and pulsating, it implies *right heart failure*. Look for the other signs, i.e. pitting oedema and large tender liver. Sometimes the JVP is so raised it can be missed, except that the ears waggle.

Dilated neck veins with no pulsation suggest *non-cardiac obstruction* (e.g. carcinoma bronchus causing superior caval obstruction or a kinked external jugular vein).

If the venous pressure rises on inspiration (it normally falls), *constrictive pericarditis* or *pericardial effusion* causing *tamponade* must be considered.

- **Observe the character of JVP.** Try to ascertain the waveform of the JVP. It should be a double pulsation consisting of:
  - a-wave atrial contraction —ends synchronous with carotid artery pulse c
  - v-wave atrial filling—when the tricuspid valve is closed by ventricular contraction—with and just after carotid pulse.

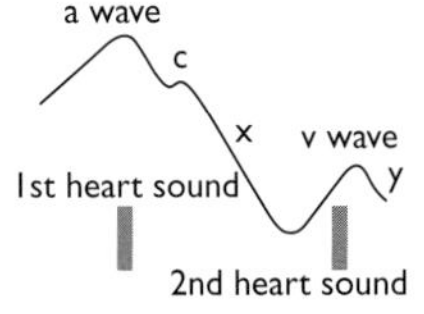

Large a waves are caused by obstruction to flow from the right atrium due to stiffness of the right ventricle from hypertrophy:

pulmonary hypertension
pulmonary stenosis
tricuspid stenosis.

Absent a wave in *atrial fibrillation*.

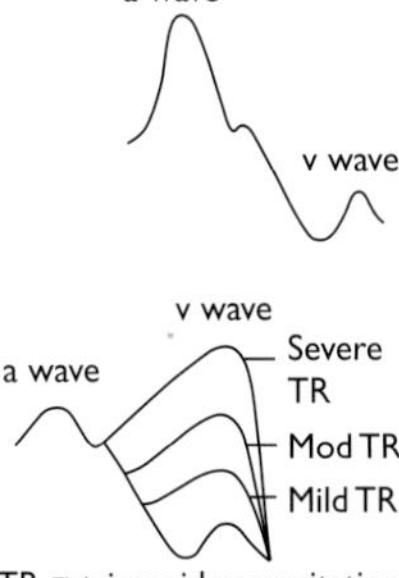

Large v waves are caused by regurgitation of blood through an *incompetent tricuspid valve* during ventricular contraction.

A sharp y descent occurs in *constrictive pericarditis*.

Cannon waves (giant a waves) occur in *complete heart block* when the right atrium occasionally contracts against a closed tricuspid valve.

The precordium

Most important, consider:

- **the apex beat**
- **heaves**
- **thrills.**

- **Inspect the precordium for abnormal pulsation**

A large left ventricle may easily be seen on the left side of the chest, sometimes in the axilla.

- **Palpate the apex beat**
  - Feel for the point furthest out and down where the pulsation can still be distinctly felt.
- **Measure the position**
  - Which space, counting down from the second space which lies below the second rib (opposite the manubriosternal angle).
  - Laterally in centimetres from the midline.
  - Describe the apex beat in relation to the mid-clavicular line, anterior axillary line and mid-axillary line.

The normal position of the apex beat is in the fifth left intercostal space on the mid clavicular line.

- **Assess character**

Try to judge if an enlarged heart is:

- **feeble** (dilated) or
- **stronger** than usual (left or right ventricle hypertrophy or both).

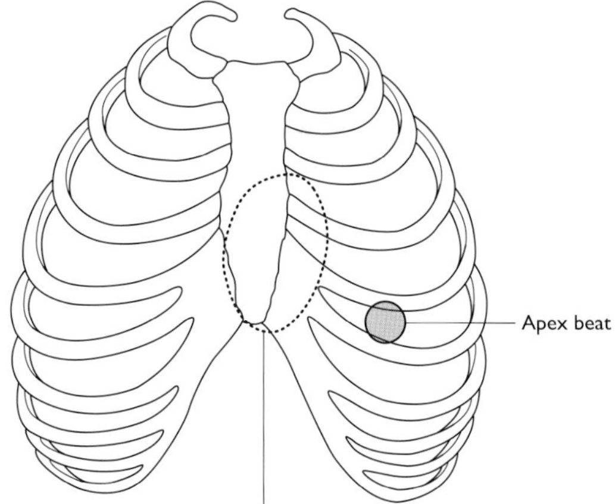

- **Thrusting displaced apex beat** occurs with volume overload: an active, large stroke volume ventricle, e.g. *mitral* or *aortic incompetence*, *left-to-right shunt* or *cardiomyopathy*.
- **Sustained apex beat** occurs with pressure overload in *aortic stenosis* and *gross hypertension*. Stroke volume is normal or reduced.
- **Tapping apex beat** (palpable first heart sound) occurs in *mitral stenosis*.
- **Diffuse pulsation asynchronous with apex beat** occurs with a *left ventricular aneurysm*—a dyskinetic apex beat.
- **Impalpable**—obesity, overinflated chest due to COPD, pericardial effusion.

- **Palpate firmly the left border of the sternum**
  - Use the flat of your hand.

A heave suggests *right ventricular hypertrophy*.

- **Palpate all over the precordium with the flat of hand for thrills (palpable murmurs).**

N.B. If by now you have found an abnormality in the cardiovascular system, think of possible causes before you listen.

For example, if left ventricle is forceful:

- Hypertension—was blood pressure (BP) raised?
- Aortic stenosis or incompetence—was pulse character normal? Will there be a murmur?
- Mitral incompetence—will there be a murmur?
- Thyrotoxicosis or anaemia.

If atrial fibrillation: is there mitral stenosis?

Auscultation

- **Listen over the four main areas of the heart** and in each area concentrate in order on:
  - **heart sounds**
  - **added sounds**
  - **murmurs.**

Keep to this order when listening or describing what you have heard, or you will miss or forget important findings.

The four main areas are:

- **apex, mitral area; 5th intercostal space, mid-clavicular line** (and axilla if there is a murmur)
- **tricuspid area; 4th intercostal space, left sternal edge**
- **aortic area; 2nd intercostal space, right sternal edge** (and neck if there is a murmur)
- **pulmonary area; 2nd intercostal space, left sternal edge.**

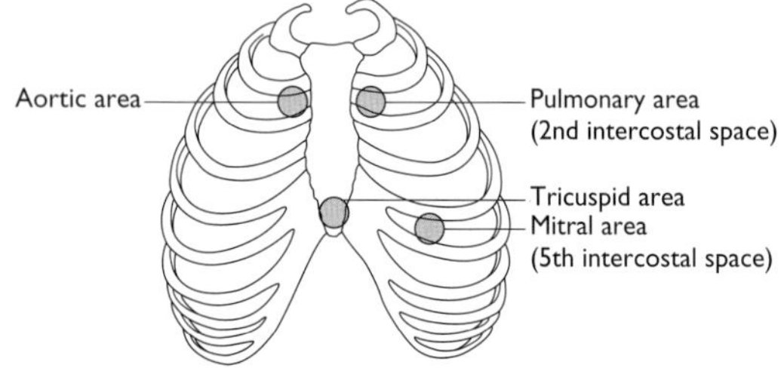

These areas represent where one hears heart sounds and murmurs associated with these valves. They do not represent the surface markings of the valves.

If you hear little, turn the patient half left, and listen over apex (having palpated for it).

The diaphragm filters out low-frequency sounds, so the bell should be used for mitral stenosis.

You may find it helpful to try to imitate what you think you hear.

Normal heart sounds

- **I Sudden cessation of mitral and tricuspid flow due to valve closure**
  - loud in *mitral stenosis*
  - soft in *mitral incompetence, aortic stenosis, left bundle-branch block*
  - variable in *complete heart block and atrial fibrillation*.
- **II Sudden cessation of aortic and pulmonary flow due to valve closure**—usually split (see below)
  - loud in *hypertension*
  - soft in *aortic* or *pulmonary stenosis*
  - wide normal split—*right bundle-branch block*
  - wide fixed split—*atrial septal defect*.

Added sounds

- **III Rapid ventricular filling sound in early diastole**

Often **normal** until about 30 years, then probably means *heart failure, fibrosed ventricle* or *constrictive pericarditis*.

- **IV Atrial contraction inducing ventricular filling towards the end of the diastole**

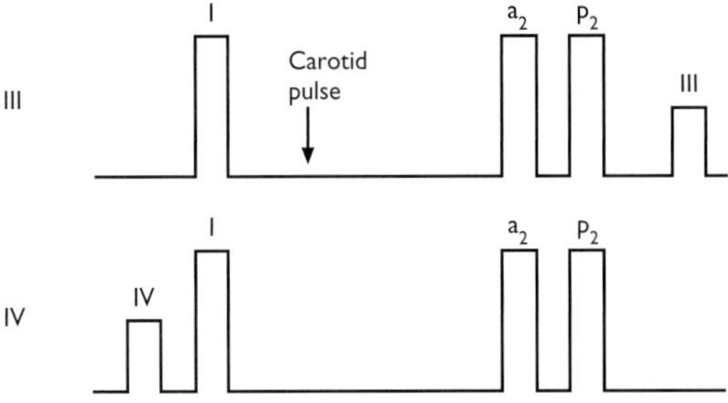

May be normal under age 20 and in athletes, but suggests increased atrial load. Not as serious a prognosis as a third heart sound.

Canter rhythm (often termed **gallop**) with tachycardia gives the following cadences:

III: Tum—te—tum or **K**en—**t**uc**k**y (k = first heart sound)

IV: te–Tum—te or **T**enne—**ss**ee (n = first heart sound)

- *Opening snap*
  - Mitral valve normally opens silently after second heart sound.
  - In *mitral stenosis*, sudden movement of rigid valve makes a click, after second heart sound (Figure 3.3).

- *Ejection click*
  - Aortic valve normally opens silently.
  - In *aortic stenosis* or *sclerosis*, can open with a click after first heart sound.

Splitting of second heart sound

Ask patients to take deep breaths in and out. Blood is drawn into the thorax during inspiration and then on to the right ventricle. There is temporarily more blood in the right ventricle than the left ventricle, and the right ventricle takes fractionally longer to empty.

Splitting is best heard during the first two or three beats of inspiration. **Do not** ask the patient to **hold** their breath in or out when assessing splitting.

Paradoxical splitting occurs in *aortic stenosis* and *left bundle-branch block*.

In both these conditions (Figure 3.4) the left ventricle takes longer to empty, thus delaying $\mathbf{a_2}$ until after $\mathbf{p_2}$. During inspiration $\mathbf{p_2}$ occurs later and the sounds draw closer together.

Murmurs

Use the diaphragm of the stethoscope for most high-pitched sounds or murmurs (e.g. aortic incompetence) and the bell for low-pitched murmurs (e.g. mitral stenosis). Note the following.

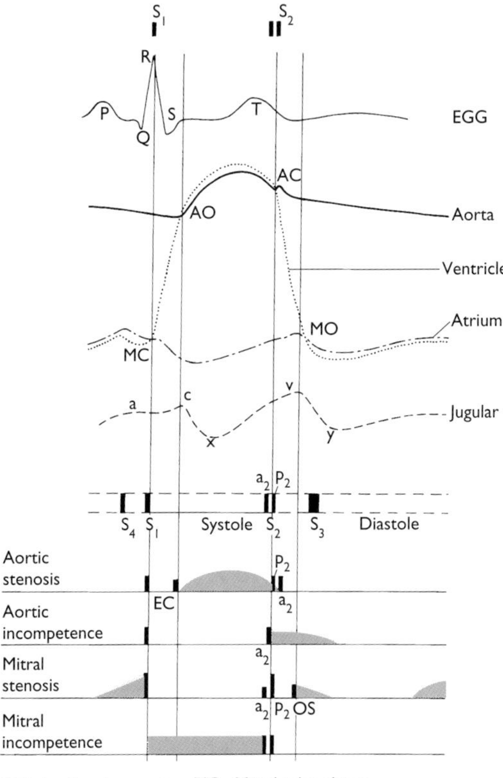

AO	Aortic valve opens	MC	Mitral valve closes
AC	Aortic valve closes	EC	Ejection click
MO	Mitral valve opens	OS	Opening snap

Figure 3.3 Relation of murmurs to pressure changes and valve movements.

- **Timing systolic or diastolic** (compare with finger on carotid pulse) (Figure 3.3).
- **Site and radiation**, for example:
  - mitral incompetence → axilla
  - aortic stenosis → carotids and apex
  - aortic incompetence → sternum.

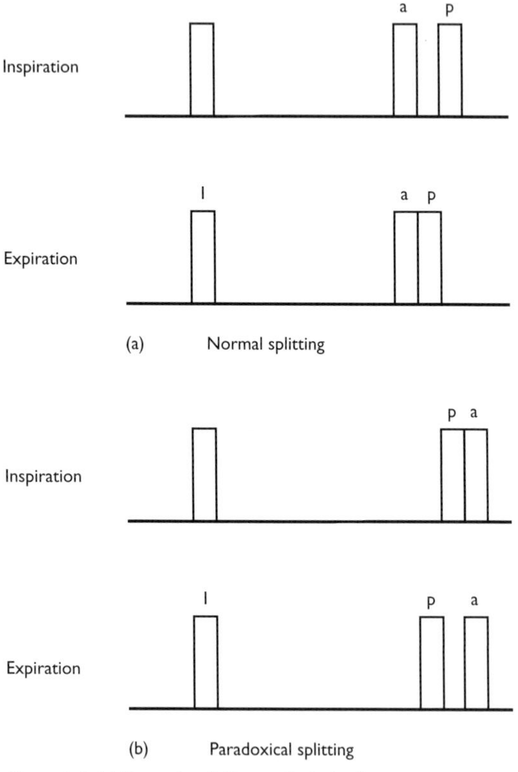

Figure 3.4 (a) Normal and (b) paradoxical splitting.

- **Character**
  - loud or soft
  - pitch, e.g. squeaking or rumbling, 'scratchy' = pericardial or pleural
  - length
    - pansystolic, throughout systole
    - early diastolic, e.g. aortic or pulmonary incompetence
    - mid systolic, e.g. aortic stenosis or flow murmur
    - mid diastolic, e.g. mitral stenosis.

- **Relation to posture**
  - sit forward—aortic incompetence louder
  - lie left side—mitral stenosis louder.
- **Relation to respiration**
  - inspiration increases the murmur of a right heart lesion
  - expiration increases the murmur of a left heart lesion
  - variable—pericardial rub.
- **Relation to exercise**
  - increases the murmur of mitral stenosis.

Optimal position for hearing murmurs

(Figure 3.5)

- **Mitral stenosis**—the patient lies on left side, arm above head; listen with bell at apex. Murmur is louder after exercise, e.g. repeated touching of toes from lying position that increases cardiac output.
- **Aortic incompetence**—the patient sits forward after deep inspiration; listen with diaphragm at lower left sternal edge.

N.B. Murmurs alone do not make the diagnosis. Take other signs into consideration, e.g. arterial or venous pulses, blood pressure, apex or heart sounds.

Loudness is often not proportional to severity of disease, and in some situations length of murmur is more important, e.g. mitral stenosis.

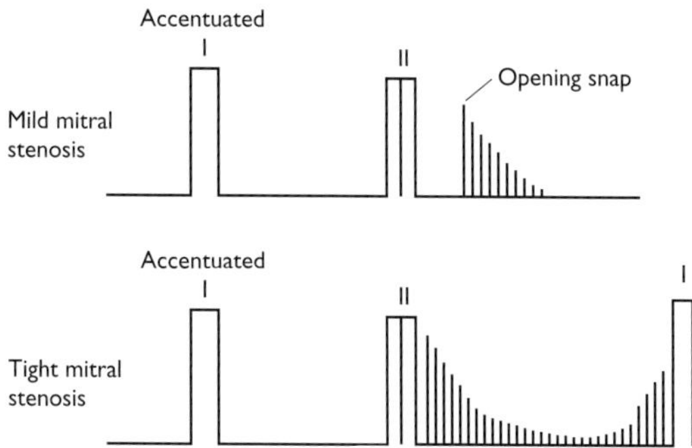

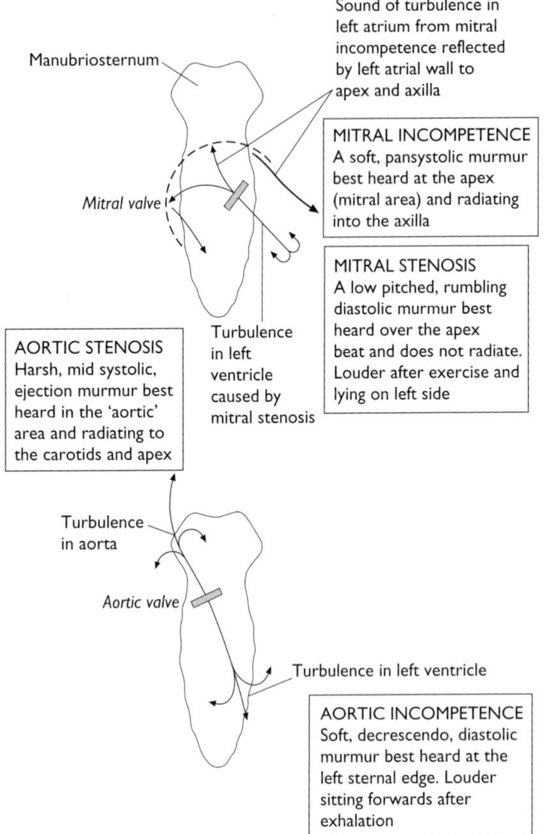

Figure 3.5 Radiation of sound from turbulent blood flow.

- For completion:
  - **auscultate base of lungs** for crepitations from left ventricular failure
  - **peripheral pulses** (palpate and listen for bruits)
  - **palpate liver**—smooth, tender, enlarged in right heart failure
  - **peripheral oedema**—ankle/sacral.

Summary of timing of murmurs

- *Ejection systolic murmur*
  - *aortic stenosis* or *sclerosis* (same murmur, due to stiffness of valve cusps and aortic walls, with normal pulse pressure). *Aortic sclerosis* is present in 50% of 50-year-olds
  - *pulmonary stenosis*
  - *atrial septal defect*
  - *Fallot's syndrome*—right outflow tract obstruction

- *Pansystolic murmur*
  - *mitral regurgitation*
  - *tricuspid regurgitation*
  - *ventricular septal defect*

- *Late systolic murmur*
  - *mitral valve prolapse* (click–murmur syndrome)
  - *hypertrophic cardiomyopathy*
  - *coarction aorta* (extending in diastole to a 'machinery murmur')

- *Early diastolic murmur*
  - *aortic regurgitation*
  - *pulmonary regurgitation*
  - Graham Steell murmur in *pulmonary hypertension* (see under Summary of common illnesses)

- *Mid–late diastolic murmur*
  - *mitral stenosis*
  - *tricuspid stenosis*
  - Austin Flint murmur in *aortic incompetence* (see under Summary of common illnesses)
  - *left atrial myxoma* (variable—can also give other murmurs)

Signs of left and right ventricular failure

Left heart failure

- dyspnoea
- basal crepitations
- fourth heart sound, or third in older patients

- Sit the patient forward and listen at the bases of the lungs with the diaphragm of the stethoscope for fine crepitations.

 Fine crepitations are caused by alveoli opening on inspiration. When a patient has been recumbent for a while, alveoli tend to collapse in the normal lung. On taking a deep breath crepitations will be heard but do not mean pulmonary oedema. Ask the patient to cough. If crepitations continue after this, pulmonary oedema may be present.

Right heart failure
  - raised JVP
  - enlarged tender liver (see later)
  - pitting oedema
- With the patient sitting forward, look for swelling over the sacral area. If there is swelling, push your thumb into the swelling and see if you leave an indentation. If you do, this is called pitting oedema.
- Check both ankles for pitting oedema.

 Oedema (fluid) collects at the most dependent part of the body. A patient who is mostly sitting will have ankle oedema, while a patient who is lying will have predominantly sacral oedema.

Functional result

- Having ascertained the basic pathology (e.g. *myocardial infarction*, *aortic stenosis*, *pericarditis*), make an assessment of the functional result.
  - **History**—how far can the patient walk, etc.
  - **Examination**—evidence of:
    - cardiac enlargement (hypertrophy or dilatation)
    - heart failure
    - arrhythmias
    - pulmonary hypertension
    - cyanosis
    - endocarditis.
  - **Investigations**—for example:
    - troponin
    - chest X-ray

- electrocardiogram (ECG)
- treadmill exercise test with ECG for ischaemia
- echocardiograph—sonar 'radar' of heart, for muscle and ventricle size, muscle contractility and ejection fraction, valve function
- 24-hour ECG tape for arrhythmias
- cardiac catheterisation for pressure measurements, blood oxygenation and angiogram
- radionucleotide scan—to image live, ischaemic or dead cardiac muscle.

Summary of common illnesses

Mitral stenosis

- small pulse—fibrillating?
- JVP only raised if heart failure
- RV_{++} LVo tapping apex
- loud I; loud p_2 if pulmonary hypertension
- opening snap (os)
- mid-diastolic murmur at apex only (low-pitched rumbling)
  - severity indicated by early opening snap and long murmur
  - best heard with the patient in left lateral position, in expiration with the stethoscope bell, particularly after exercise has increased cardiac output
  - presystolic accentuation of murmur (absent if atrial fibrillation and stiff cusps)
- sounds 'ta ta rooofoo T' from II os murmur I

Mitral incompetence

- fibrillating?
- JVP only raised if heart failure
- RV_{+} LV_{++} systolic thrill
- soft I; loud p_2 if pulmonary hypertension
- pansystolic murmur apex → axilla

Mitral valve prolapse

- mid-systolic click, late systolic murmur
  - posterior cusp—murmur apex → axilla
  - anterior cusp—murmur apex → aortic area

There are three stages:

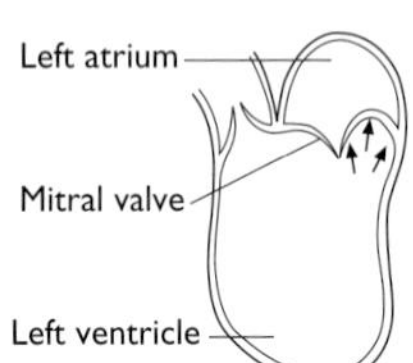

Click from billowing of cusp – larger than other cusp – may occur in 10% of females

Heard best on standing

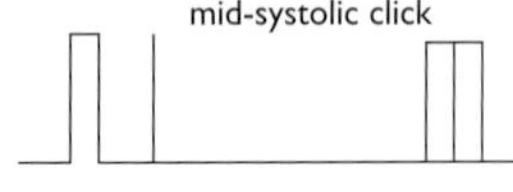

Click/late systolic murmur. After 'click', prolapsing cusp allows regurgitation

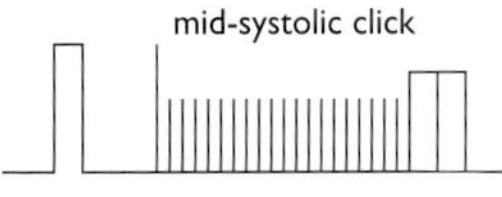

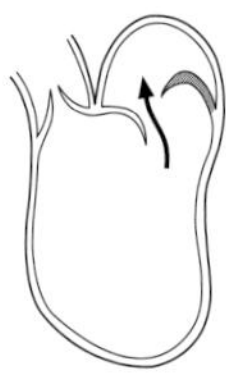

Cusp flails giving pansystolic regurgitation

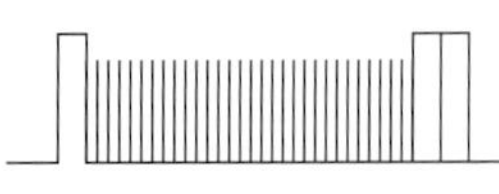

Aortic stenosis

- plateau pulse—narrow pulse pressure
- JVP only raised if heart failure
- LV_{++} systolic thrill
- soft a_2 with paradoxical split (± ejection click)
- harsh mid-systolic murmur, apex and base, radiating to carotids
  - note discrepancy of forceful apex and feeble arterial pulse
  - the longer the murmur, the tighter the stenosis. Loudness does not necessarily imply severity

Aortic incompetence

- water-hammer pulse—wide pulse pressure. Pulse visible in carotids

- JVP only raised if heart failure
- LV_{++} with dilation
- (ejection click)
- early diastolic murmur base → lower sternum (also ejection systolic murmur from increased flow)
  - (sometimes Austin Flint murmur—see below)
  - heard best with patient leaning forward, in expiration
  - the longer the murmur, the more severe the regurgitation

Tricuspid incompetence

- JVP large V wave
- RV_{++}, no thrill
- soft pansystolic murmur at maximal tricuspid area
- increases on inspiration

Austin Flint murmur

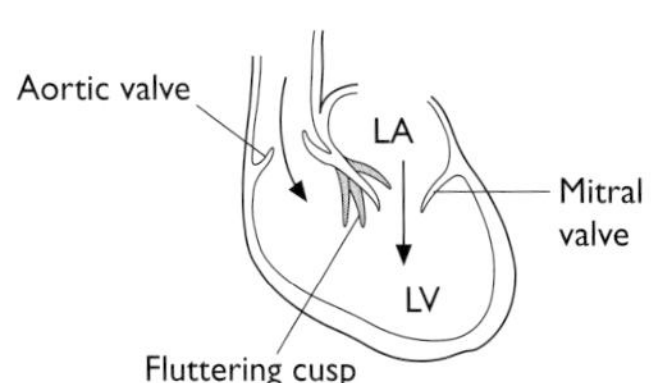

- mid-diastolic murmur (like mitral stenosis) in aortic incompetence due to regurgitant stream of blood on anterior cusp mitral valve

Graham Steell murmur

- pulmonary early diastolic murmur (functional pulmonary incompetence) in mitral stenosis or other causes of pulmonary hypertension

Atrial septal defect

- JVP only raised if failure or tricuspid incompetence
- RV_{++} LVo

- widely fixed split-second sound
- pulmonary systolic murmur (tricuspid diastolic flow murmur)

Ventricular septal defect

- RV_+ LV_+
- pansystolic murmur on left sternal edge (loud if small defect)

Patent ductus arteriosus

- systolic → diastolic 'machinery' or continuous murmur below left clavicle

Metal prosthetic valves

- loud clicks with short flow murmur
  - aortic systolic
  - mitral diastolic
- need anticoagulation

Tissue prosthetic valves

- porcine xenograft or human homograft
- tend to fibrose after 7–10 years, leading to stenosis and incompetence
- may not require anticoagulation

Pericardial rub

- scratchy, superficial noise heard in systole and diastole
- brought out by stethoscope pressure, and sometimes variable with respiration

Infectious endocarditis (diagnosis made from blood cultures)

- febrile, unwell, anaemia
- clubbing
- splinter haemorrhages
- Osler's nodes
- cardiac murmur
- splenomegaly
- haematuria

Rheumatic fever

- flitting arthralgia
- erythema nodosum or erythema marginatum
- tachycardia
- murmurs
- *Sydenham's chorea* (irregular, uncontrollable jerks of limbs, tongue)

Clues to diagnosis from facial appearance

- *Down's syndrome* from 21 trisomy
  - ventricular septal defect
  - patent ductus arteriosus
- *thyrotoxicosis*—atrial fibrillation
- *myxoedema* from hypothyroid—cardiomyopathy
- dusky, congested face—*superior vena cava obstruction*
- red cheeks in infra-orbital region in mitral facies from mitral stenosis

Clues to diagnosis from general appearance

- *Turner's syndrome* from sex chromosomes XO
  - female, short stature, web of neck
  - coarctation of aorta
- *Marfan's syndrome*
  - tall patient with long, thin fingers
  - aortic regurgitation

Peripheral arteries

- **Feel all peripheral pulses** (Figure 3.6). Lower-limb pulses are usually felt after examining the abdomen.

Diminished or absent pulses suggest *arterial stenosis* or *occlusion*.

The lower-limb pulses are particularly important if there is a history of *intermittent claudication*.

Auscultation of the carotid and femoral vessels is useful if there is a suspicion these arteries are stenosed. A bruit is heard if the stenosis causes turbulent flow.

Coarctation of the aorta delays the femoral pulse after the radial pulse.

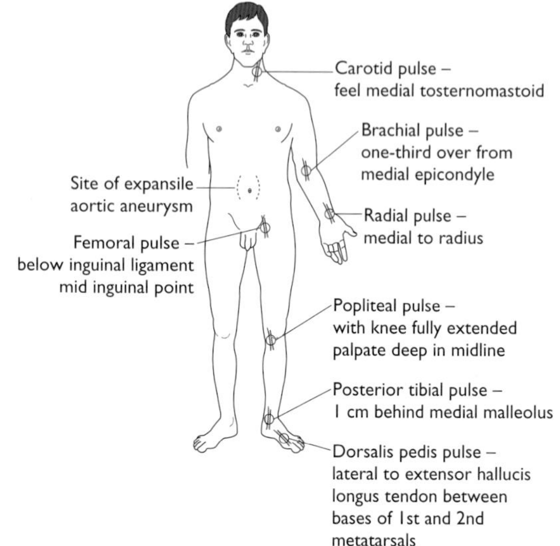

Figure 3.6 Sites of peripheral pulses.

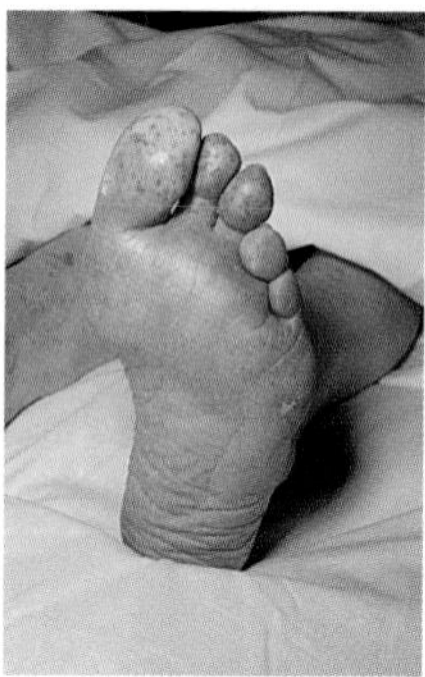

Figure 3.7 Ischaemic toes from acute arterial insufficiency—white toes becoming blue, with erythematous reaction at demarcation.

Peripheral vascular disease

- white or blue discoloration (Figure 3.7)
- ulcers with little granulation tissue and slow healing
- shiny skin, loss of hairs, thickened dystrophic nails

- absent pulses
- Buerger's test of severity of arterial insufficiency
  - loss of autoregulation of blood flow
  - patient lying supine, lift leg up to 45°—positive test: pallor of foot; venous guttering
  - hang legs over side of bed: note time to capillary and venous filling; reactive hyperaemia; subsequent cyanosis

Diabetes, when present, also signs from **neuropathy**:

- dry skin with thickened epidermis
- callus from increased foot pressure over abnormal sites, e.g. under tarsal heads in mid-foot, secondary to motor neuropathy and change in distribution of weight (Figure 3.8)
- absent ankle reflexes
- decreased sensation

Aortic aneurysm

- central abdominal pulsation visible or palpable
- need to distinguish from normal, palpable aorta in midline in thin people
  - aortic aneurysm is expansible to each side as well as forwards
  - a bruit may be audible
  - associated with femoral and popliteal artery aneurysms

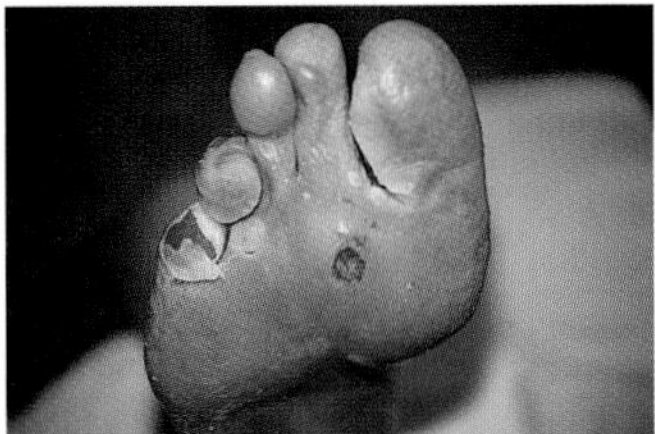

Figure 3.8 Diabetic foot—shiny, dry skin with ulcer from abnormal pressure point from motor neuropathy and painless, unsuspected blister on toe.

Varicose veins

- Varicose veins and herniae (see Chapter 5) are examined **when the patient is standing**, possibly at the end of the whole examination at the same time as the gait (see Chapter 2).

Majority are associated with incompetent valves in the long saphenous vein or short saphenous vein:
- long saphenous—from femoral vein in groin to medial side of lower leg
- short saphenous—from popliteal fossa to back of calf and lateral malleolus.

- **Observe (Figure 3.9):**
  - swelling
  - pigmentation } indicate chronic venous insufficiency
  - eczema } indicate chronic venous insufficiency
  - inflammation—suggests thrombophlebitis
- **Palpate:**
  - soft or hard (thrombosed)
  - tender—thrombophlebitis
  - cough impulse—implies incompetent valves

Incompetent valves can be confirmed by the **Trendelenburg test**:

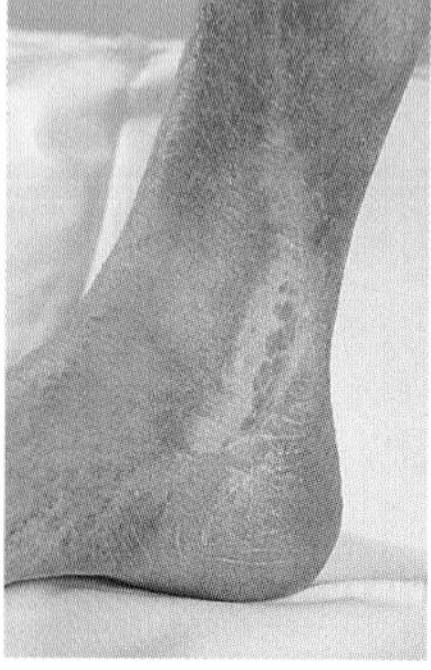

Figure 3.9 Healing varicose ulcer—classic site in lower leg medially with pigmentation from venous stasis.

- Elevate leg to empty veins.
- Occlude long saphenous vein with a tourniquet around upper thigh.
- Stand patient up.
- If veins fill rapidly, this indicates incompetent thigh perforators below the tourniquet.
- If, after release of tourniquet, veins fill rapidly, this indicates incompetent saphenofemoral junction.

If veins fill immediately on standing, then incompetent valves are in thigh or calf, so do the **Perthes test**:

- As for Trendelenburg, but on standing let some blood enter veins by temporary release of groin pressure.
- Ask patient to stand up and down on toes.
- Veins become less tense if:
  - muscle pump is satisfactory
  - perforating calf veins are patent with competent valves.

System-oriented examination

'Examine the cardiovascular system'

- hands—splinter haemorrhages
- radial pulse—rate, rhythm, waveform, volume, state of artery
- waveform and volume best examined at the brachial or carotid artery
- *'I would normally measure the blood pressure now; would you like me to do so?'*
- eyes—anaemia
- tongue—central cyanosis
- JVP—height, waveform
- apex beat—site, character
- auscultate
  - at apex (with thumb on carotid artery for timing)
    - heart sounds
    - added sounds
    - murmurs
  - in neck over carotid artery—each area of precordium with diaphragm
    - aortic incompetence—lean forward in full expiration with diaphragm

- mitral stenosis—lie patient on left side and listen at apex with bell

- *'I would normally now listen to the bases for crepitations, examine for hepatomegaly, peripheral oedema and peripheral pulses. Would you like me to do so?'*

CHAPTER 4
Examination of the chest

General inspection

- **Examine the patient for:**
  - signs of respiratory distress—use of accessory muscles, on oxygen therapy, inspect sputum pot from the end of the bed
  - **nicotine** on fingers
  - **clubbing**: respiratory causes include:
    - *carcinoma of bronchus*
    - *mesothelioma*
    - *bronchiectasis*
    - *lung abscess*
    - *empyema*
    - *fibrosing alveolitis*
  - **evidence of respiratory failure:**
    - **hypoxia**: central cyanosis
    - **hypercapnia**: drowsiness, confusion, dilated pupils, papilloedema, warm hands, bounding pulse, dilated veins, coarse tremor/flap
  - **respiratory rate**: count per minute or for 30 seconds and multiply by 2
  - **pattern of respiration**: **Cheyne–Stokes**:
    - alternating hyperventilation and apnoea
    - severe increased intracranial pressure
    - left ventricular failure
    - high altitude
  - **obstructive airways disease**:
    - pursed-lip breathing:

Clinical Skills and Examination: The Core Curriculum. By R Turner, B Angus, A Handa, C Hatton. ©2009 Blackwell Publishing, ISBN: 9781405157513.

expiration against partially closed lips
chronic obstructive airways disease to delayed closure of bronchioles

- use of accessory muscles:

- sternomastoids
- strap muscles and platysmus

- **wheezing**
- **stridor**: partial obstruction of major airway
- **hoarse voice**:
  - abnormal vocal cords
    or *recurrent laryngeal palsy*.

First examine the front of the chest fully and then similarly examine the back of the chest.

Inspection of the chest

- **Rest the patient comfortably in the bed at 45°**
  - distended neck, puffy blue face and arms
  - superior mediastinal obstruction.
- **Inspect the shape of the chest**
  - asymmetry: diminution of one side
    - lung collapse
    - fibrosis
  - deformity: check spine
  - pectus excavatum: sunken sternum
  - scars

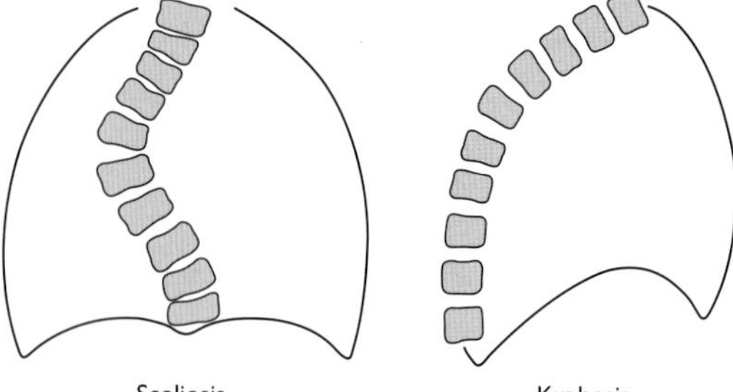

- **obstructive airways disease**
  - barrel chest: lower costal recession on deep inspiration. Cricoid cartilage close to sternal notch. Chest appears to be fixed in inspiration.

Palpation

- **Check mediastinum position**
  - **trachea**—check position: palpate with a single finger in the midline and determine if it slips preferentially to one side or the other.

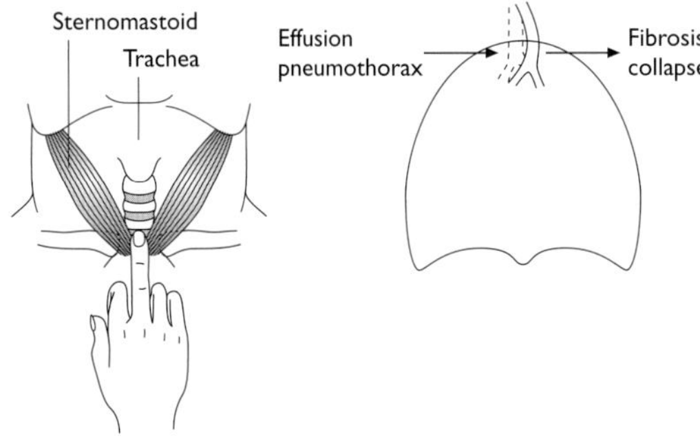

- **Lymph nodes,** supraclavicular fossae/axillae—*tuberculosis, lymphoma, cancer of the bronchus.*
- **Apex beat** may be displaced because of enlarged heart and not a shift in the mediastinum.
- **Unequal movement of chest.**
  - Classic method of palpation:
    - extend your fingers—anchor fingertips far laterally around chest wall so your extended thumbs meet in midline

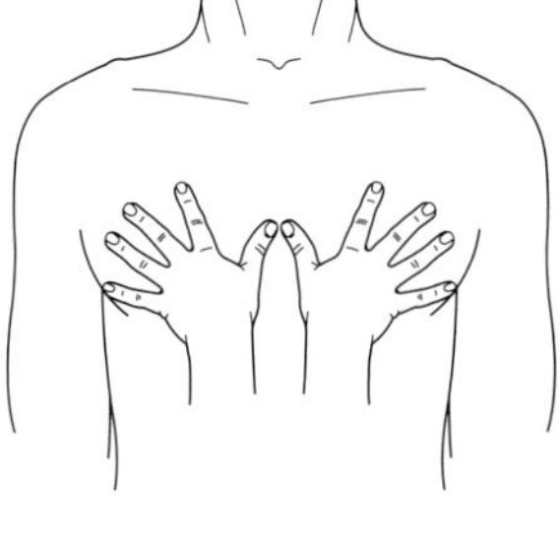

    - on inspiration, assess whether asymmetrical movement of thumbs from midline.

- Alternative method of palpation:
  - lay a hand comfortably on either side of the chest and, using these as a gauge, assess if there is diminution of movement on one side during inspiration.

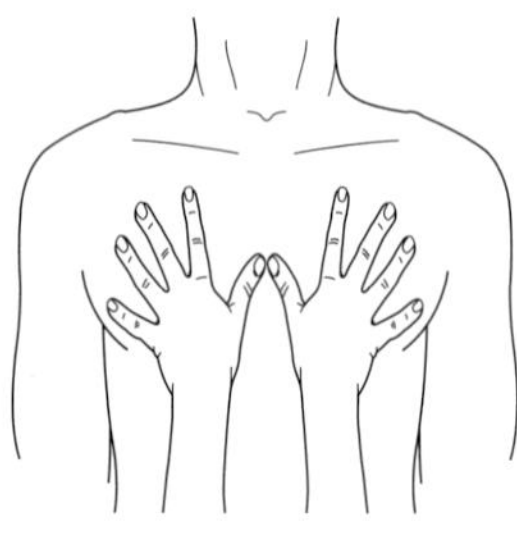

N.B. Diminution of movement on one side indicates pathology on that side.

Percussion

- Percuss with the middle finger of one hand against the middle phalanx of the middle finger of the other, laid flat on the chest. The finger should strike at right angles. Practise percussion whenever possible.
- **Percuss both sides of the chest for resonance**, at top, middle and lower segments. Compare sides, and if different also compare the front and back of chest.
- If a dull area exists, map out its limits by percussing from a resonant to the dull area.
- Percuss the level of the diaphragm from above downwards.

Increased resonance may occur in:

- *pneumothorax*
- *emphysema*.

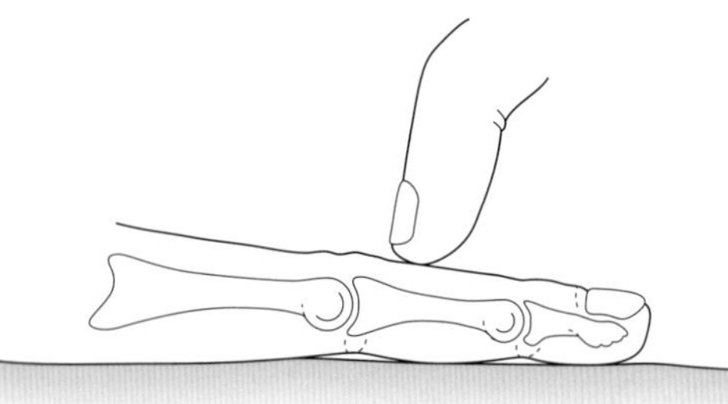

Decreased resonance may occur in:

- *effusion:* very dull—sometimes called stony dullness
- *solid lung*
  - consolidation
  - collapse
  - abscess
- *neoplasm*.

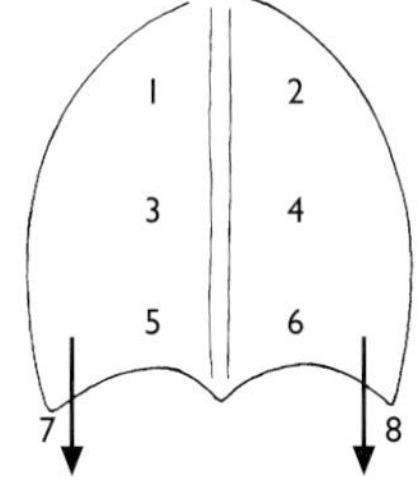

Remember the surface markings of the lungs when percussing.

The lower lobe predominates posteriorly and the upper lobe predominates anteriorly (Figure 4.1).

Auscultation

- **Before listening, ask patient to cough up any sputum** which may provide noises for bronchi.
- Use the bell of the stethoscope and listen at the top, middle and bottom of both sides of the chest, and then in the axilla.

Ask the patient to breathe through their mouth moderately deeply. It helps to demonstrate this yourself.

The stethoscope diaphragm is less effective if the patient is thin with prominent ribs or if the chest is hairy.

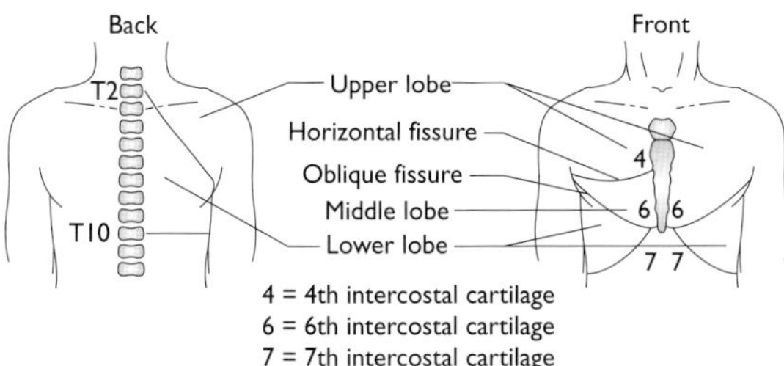

Figure 4.1 Percuss the diaphragm from above downwards. These markings are at full inspiration. Under normal examination conditions the hepatic dullness extends to the fifth intercostal cartilage.

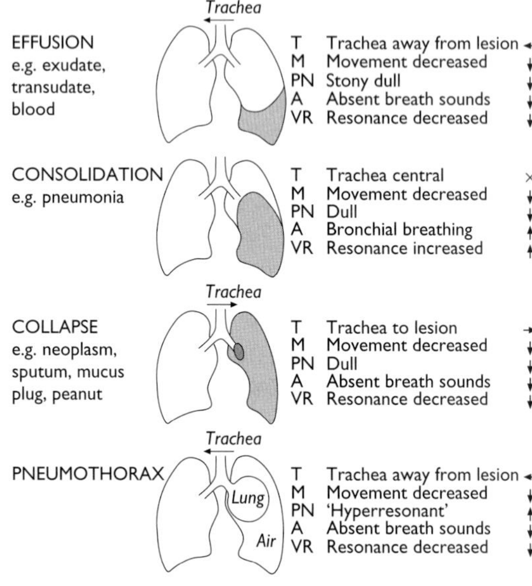

Figure 4.2 Auscultation.

- **Listen for breath sounds,** comparing both sides (Figure 4.2):
  - **vesicular:** normal breath sounds

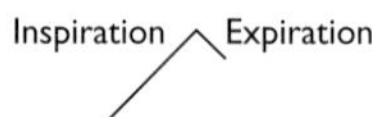

  - **bronchial:** patent bronchi plus conducting tissue

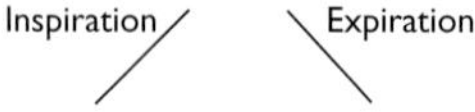

  - sounds similar to sounds with stethoscope over trachea

consolidation (usually pneumonia)
neoplasm
fibrosis
abscess

not collapse, effusion (except commonly at the top of an effusion)

- **diminution**: indicates either no air movement (e.g. obstructed bronchus) or air or fluid preventing sound conduction

effusion
pneumothorax
emphysema
collapse.

- **Listen for added sounds,** and note if inspiratory or expiratory:

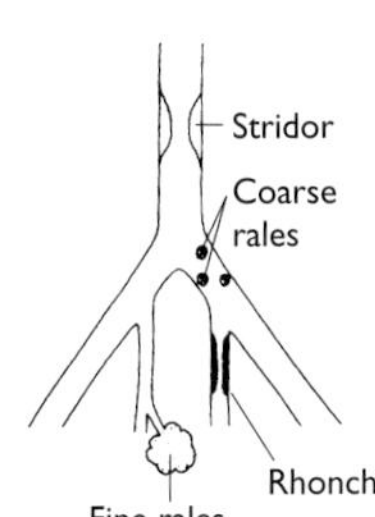

  - **pleural rub**: caused by *pleurisy* (inflammation due to infection or infarction), but make sure it does not come from friction of skin or hairs against stethoscope
  - **rhonchi or wheezing**: constricted air passages giving dry tubular sounds, often maximal on expiration
  - **râles or crepitations** or crackles:
    - fine—*heart failure* or *alveolitis*
    - medium—*infection*
    - coarse—air bubbling through fluid in larger bronchioles, e.g. *bronchiectasis*. If relieved by coughing, suggests from bronchioles.

Vocal resonance

Normally only done if pathology is suspected, but you must practise to become familiar with normal resonance.

- **Ask the patient to repeat '99'** while listening to chest in the same areas as auscultation. The sounds are louder over areas of consolidation. Compare both sides.

At the surface of an *effusion* the words '99' take on a bleating character like a goat, which is called **aegophony**. If vocal resonance is gross, **whispering pectoriloquy** can be elicited by asking the patient to ***whisper*** '1, 2, 3, 4'.

N.B. Vocal fremitus, breath sounds and vocal resonance all depend on the same criteria and vary together.

To determine further clues check:

- chest movement asymmetry
- mediastinum displacement
- percussion.

Sputum

Bedside examination of the sputum is unpleasant but important.

- Look for:
  - **quantity** (increased grossly in bronchiectasis)
  - **consistency** (if all mucus, it may be saliva)
  - **colour** (if yellow or green it may be infected)
  - **blood**—*cancer, tuberculosis, embolus.*

Functional result

- Make an assessment of the functional result.
  - **History**—how far can the patient walk, etc.
  - **Examination**:
    - $P\text{O}_2$¬: central cyanosis; confusion
    - $P\text{CO}_2$↑: peripheral signs
      - warm periphery
      - dilated veins
      - bounding pulse
      - flapping tremor

      central signs
      - drowsy
      - papilloedema
      - small pupils
    - check by arterial blood gases
  - **Tests** (usually of obstructive airways disease) at the bedside:
    - **Expiration time**: an assessment of airways obstruction can be made by timing the period of full expiration through wide-open mouth following a deep breath. This should be less than 2 seconds when normal.

- **Chest expansion**: expansion from full inspiration to full expiration should be more than 5 cm. Reduced if hyperinflation of the chest is due to chronic obstructive airways disease.
- **Peak flow meter**: a measure of airways obstruction is the peak rate of flow of air out of the lungs. A record is made using a machine and repeating for the 'best of three'. Normal 300–500 l/min.

Summary of common illnesses

Asthma

- patient distressed, tachypnoeic, unable to talk easily
- wheeze on expiration audible or by auscultation but beware of a silent chest
- overinflated chest with hyperresonance
- if central cyanosis: critically ill, artificial ventilation?
- pulsus paradoxus (may be normal between attacks and rarely measured)
- often due to atopy
- enquire about exposure to antigens:
  - house dust mite
  - cats or dogs

Obstructive airways disease (chronic)

- barrel chest
- accessory muscles of respiration in use
- hyperresonance
- depressed diaphragm—indrawing lower costal margin on inspiration
- diminished breath sounds:
  - **blue bloater**:

central cyanosis
signs of carbon dioxide retention
obese
not dyspnoeic
ankle oedema: may or may not have right heart failure

- **pink puffer:**

  not cyanosed
  no carbon dioxide retention
  thin
  dyspnoeic
  no oedema

Bronchiectasis

- clubbing
- constant green/yellow phlegm
- coarse râles over affected area
- usually due to cystic fibrosis in young patients

Fibrosing alveolitis (usual interstitial pneumonitis)

- clubbing
- fine, unexplained râles, widespread over bases

System-oriented examination

'Examine the respiration system'

- general examination from end of bed
- hands: clubbing, signs of increased carbon dioxide (warm hands, bounding pulse, coarse tremor)
- tongue: central cyanosis
- trachea
- supraclavicular nodes
- inspection
  - shape of chest
  - chest movements
  - respiration rate/distress
- palpation: unequal movement of chest using hands
- percussion: upper segments (L, R), middle (L, R) and lower segments (L, R)
- auscultation:
  - breath sounds
  - added sounds: crepitations, bronchospasm, pleural rub, stridor (vocal fremitus)
- if obstructive airways disease:
  - expiration time (see under Functional result)

CHAPTER 5

Examination of the abdomen

General inspection

- **Look for signs of**:
  - **chronic liver disease**:
    - *clubbing*
    - *leukonychia*
    - *palmar erythema*
    - *telangiectasia* on face
    - *icterus* (Figure 2.19)
    - *spider naevi* (Figure 5.1)
    - *gynaecomastia*
    - alcohol abuse

  - *Dupuytren's contracture*
  - *parotid enlargement*
  - *testicular atrophy*

  Signs of chronic liver disease are usually obvious, but we are all allowed up to six spider naevi (particularly if pregnant).

  - **liver failure**:
    - *liver flap*
    - *foetor hepaticus*
    - *confusion*
  - **anaemia**—look at conjunctiva, tongue
  - **iron deficiency**:
    - *koilonychia*
    - *smooth tongue*
    - *angular stomatitis*—can be from ill-fitting dentures or edentulous state

Clinical Skills and Examination: The Core Curriculum. By R Turner, B Angus, A Handa, C Hatton. ©2009 Blackwell Publishing, ISBN: 9781405157513.

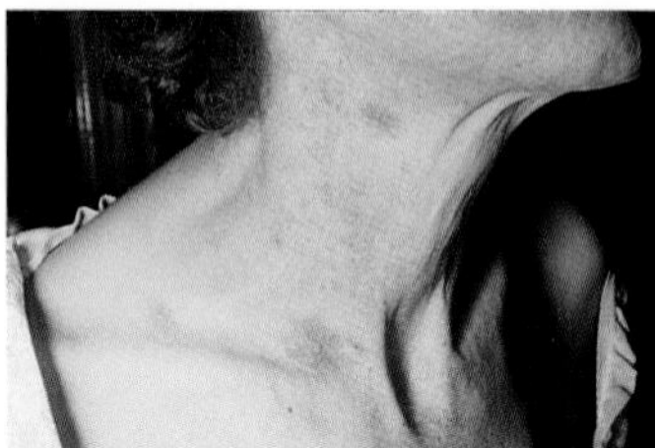

Figure 5.1 Spider naevi in cirrhosis—talangiectasia radiating from central arteriole.

- **B_{12} or folate deficiency**—'beef steak' or smooth tongue.
- **Look at lips**:
  - pale—examine conjunctivae for anaemia
    - brown freckles—*Peutz–Jeghers syndrome*—polyps in small bowel can bleed, intussuscept or become malignant.
    - telangiectasia—*Osler–Weber–Rendu syndrome*—gastrointestinal telangiectasia can bleed.
- **Look at mouth**:
  - **dry tongue**—'dehydration' or mouth-breathing

If patient seems dehydrated, lift fold of skin on neck. Skin remains raised with dehydration and old age.

- central cyanosis in chronic liver disease from pulmonary arteriovenous shunting
- *Candida*—red tongue, white patches on palate
- *gingivitis*
- ulcers
  - Crohn's disease, ulcerative colitis
  - aphthous with coeliac disease
- teeth
- breath—*ketosis*, *ethanol*, *foetor hepaticus* and *uraemia*.
- **Palpate for nodes** behind the left sternoclavicular joint.

A hard node felt behind the left sternoclavicular joint may be a **Virchow's node** and suggests an abdominal neoplasm spread by lymphatics via the thoracic duct.

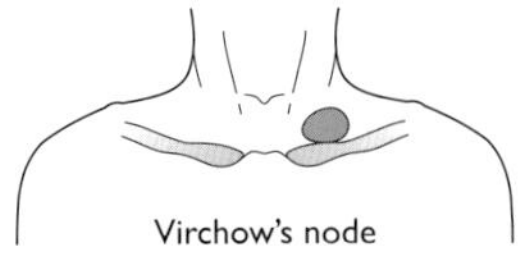

Inspection of the abdomen

- **Lie the patient flat** (one pillow) with arms by their sides.
- **Expose the abdomen** from chest (just below breasts) to groin (so that you can see the inguinal region but maintain modesty, mostly to the top of the patient's pubic hairline).

In an exam, stand back to look at the abdomen, so the examiner is impressed you are inspecting before palpating!

- **Look for**:
  - skin—striae: pink in *Cushing's syndrome*
  - body hair
  - nodules
  - surgical scars
  - swelling—central or flank
    - symmetrical or asymmetrical. May be due to:

  - flatus
  - faeces
  - fetus
  - fat
  - fluid (ascites, ovarian cyst)

  - movement: on respiration
  - peristalsis: may be visible in thin normal person
  - pulsation
  - hernia
  - dilated veins—flow of blood in vein (Figure 5.2) is:
    - **superior**: due to inferior vena cava obstruction
    - **inferior**: due to superior vena cava obstruction

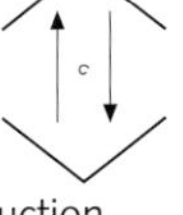

  - **radiating from navel**: due to portal vein hypertension.

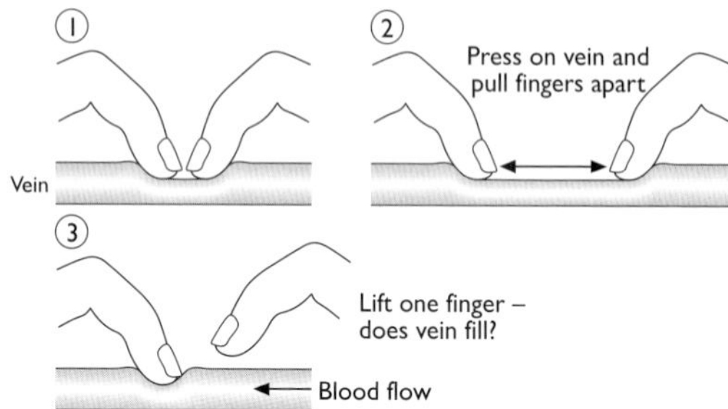

Figure 5.2 William Harvey's method of checking vein filling.

Palpation of the abdomen

- **Palpate the groins** for enlarged lymph nodes. (If you don't do it now, you may forget later!)

Most people have small, shotty nodes. Most enlarged tender nodes arise from infection in legs or feet.

If large nodes, palpate spleen carefully—lymphoma or leukaemia.

- **Before you feel the abdomen**:
  - **ask**: 'Is your tummy painful anywhere? Tell me if I hurt you.'
  - **have warm hands**, and the patient lying straight and flat, with one pillow and hands by their sides.
- **The abdomen is traditionally divided into nine areas** (see diagram below):
  - **lightly palpate each of the nine areas first**, starting away from the site of pain or tenderness. The hand should be flat on the abdomen and feel by flexing fingers at the metacarpophalangeal joints. Be gentle
  - **look at the patient's face** to see if palpation is hurting them
  - **deep palpation**. If there is no evidence of distress palpate the abdomen in the same manner repeating the nine areas but deeper.

Tenderness may be superficial, deep or rebound.

Rebound tenderness from movement of inflamed viscera of peritonitis against parietal peritoneum. First percuss

Describe findings using these descriptions:

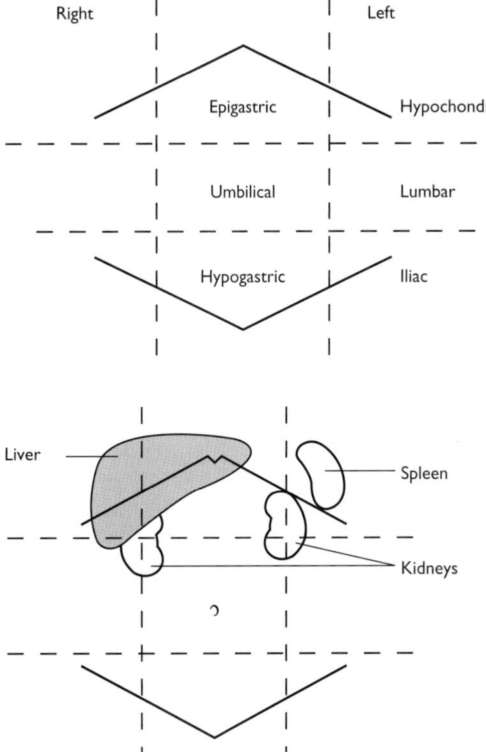

abdomen lightly, then more vigorously. If there is no pain, you can proceed to deep palpation with sudden removal of hand. Many clinicians now think that deep palpation and then suddenly letting go is very painful and unnecessarily unkind. Thus you can either try percussion or ask the patient to 'suck their tummy in and then blow it up as much as they can' to simulate rebound tenderness. This allows movement of the peritoneum and will give pain if the patient has peritoneal inflammation.

Guarding may be noted during palpation. This is a voluntary muscle spasm to protect from pain.

Rigidity. Fixed, tense abdominal muscles from reflex involuntary spasm. Occurs in generalised peritonitis.

Palpation of the organs

Liver

- **Palpate** with fingers flexed at metacarpophalangeal joints, using side of forefinger parallel with liver, with the patient breathing moderately deeply. Start in the right iliac fossa and work up towards the right costal margin.
- **Describe position of liver edge** in centimetres below the costal margin of the mid-clavicular line. Feel surface of enlarged liver and edge for:
  - **texture**
  - **regular/irregular edge**
  - **tender**
  - **pulsatile** (in tricuspid incompetence)
- **Percuss the upper and lower borders of liver** after palpation to confirm findings.

If the liver is not felt and the right hypochondrium is dull, the liver may extend to the hypogastrium. Palpate lower down.

- If the liver is large, describe:

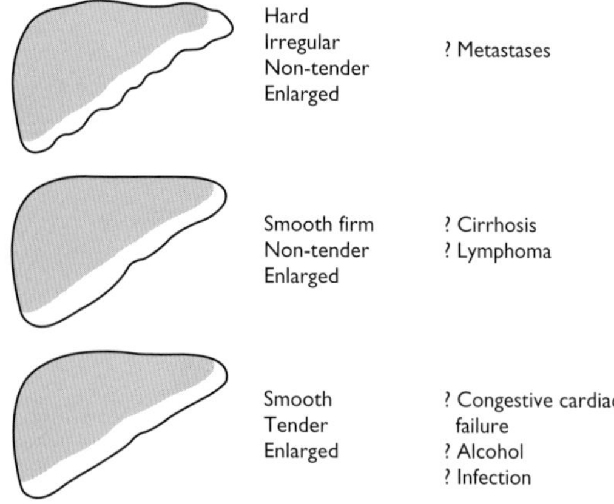

If large, remember to feel for the spleen.

Spleen

- As for the liver, **palpate** starting in the right iliac fossa and moving diagnonally towards the left costal margin in the hypochondrium.
- **Ask the patient to take a deep breath**, to bring the spleen down so it can be palpated.
- If the spleen is not palpable, **percuss** area for splenic dullness—the spleen can be enlarged to the hypogastrium.

If a slightly enlarged spleen is suspected, lie the patient on the right side with the left arm hanging loosely in front and again feel on deep inspiration or put your left hand behind the left rib cage and pull the patient towards you while palpating with your right hand in the subcostal area for the spleen.

- **Check** characteristics of the spleen:
  - **site**
  - **shape (?notch)**
  - **cannot get above it**
  - **moves on respiration**
  - **dull to percussion**.
- Describe as for liver.

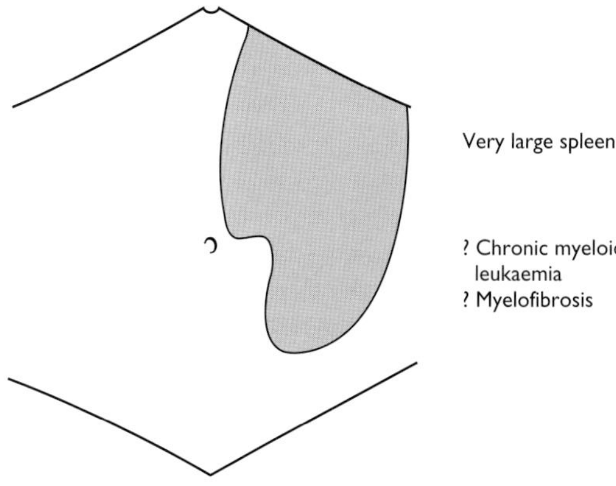

Very large spleen

? Chronic myeloid leukaemia
? Myelofibrosis

Kidneys

- **Palpate bimanually, called ballotting.**
- **Push up with left hand in renal angle** and feel kidney anteriorly with right hand.
- **Ask the patient to take a deep breath** to bring kidneys between hands.

Tenderness is common over the kidneys if there is infection. A large kidney may indicate a *tumour*, *polycystic disease* or *hydronephrosis*.

Masses

- **Carefully palpate the whole of the abdomen.** If a mass is found, describe:
  - **site**
  - **size**
  - **shape**
  - **consistency**—faeces may be indented by pressure
  - **fixation or mobility**—does it move on respiration?
  - **tender**
  - **pulsatile**—transmitted pulsation from aorta or pulsatile swelling
  - **dull to percussion**—particularly important to determine if bowel is in front of mass
  - **does it alter after defaecation or micturition?**

Aorta

- **Palpate in the midline above the umbilicus** for a pulsatile mass. If easily palpated, check if it is expansile. It is often possible to feel a normal aortic pulsation in thin individuals. However, if there is any suspicion of expansibility then suspect aortic aneurysm and proceed to ultrasonography in males over 50 and women over 60 years. May be:
  - normal aorta in a thin person
  - unfolded aorta
  - aneurysm.

Percussion

- **Dullness on percussion**:
  - ascites—free fluid
  - an organ, e.g. liver, spleen
  - tumour, e.g. *large ovarian cyst*.
- **Percuss liver, spleen and kidneys after palpation of each organ.**
- **Percuss any suspected mass.**

The midline of the abdomen should be resonant—if not, think of *gastric neoplasm, omental secondaries, enlarged bladder, ovarian cyst, pregnancy*.

- If there is generalised swelling of the abdomen, lie the patient on one side and mark the upper level of dullness. Roll the patient to the other side and see if the level shifts. This is called **shifting dullness**.

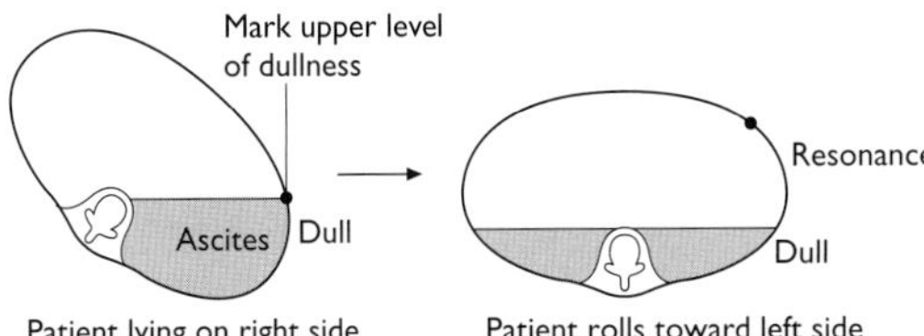

Auscultation

Bowel sounds

- Listen over the abdomen with the diaphragm of the stethoscope.

Obstruction of the bowel gives hyperactive 'tinkling' bowel sounds.

Paralytic ileus or *generalised peritonitis* give complete absence of bowel sounds.

- Listen for hepatic bruits in patients with liver disease:
  - *primary liver cell cancer*
  - *alcoholic hepatitis*
  - *acquired arteriovenous shunts* from biopsy or trauma.

Arterial bruits

If appropriate from the history or examination (e.g. hypertension), listen for bruits over the renal or femoral arteries. Renal arteries are sometimes best heard over the back.

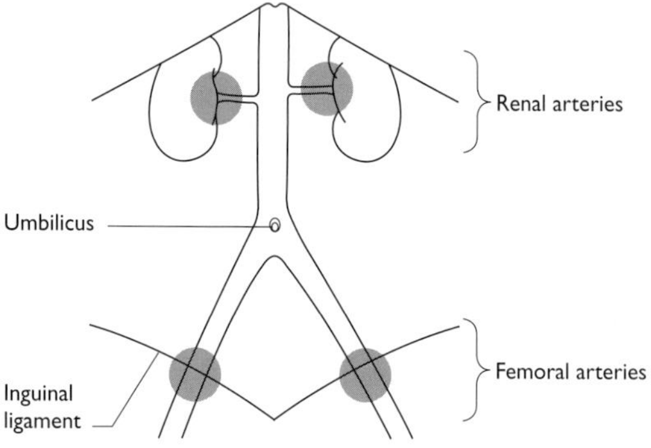

Renal artery stenosis may be the cause of hypertension.

Patients with *intermittent claudication* may have flow bruits over the femoral arteries from narrowing, e.g. *atheroma*.

Herniae

- **Establish the appropriate anatomical landmarks**—pubic tubercle, anterior superior iliac spine, femoral artery.

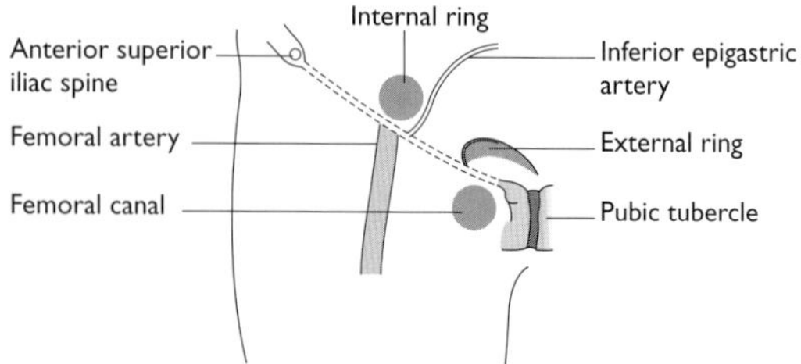

- **Examine the patient standing and ask them to cough**—enlargement of a groin swelling suggests a hernia.

Indirect inguinal hernia: swelling reduced to internal inguinal ring by pressure on contents of hernial sac and then controlled by pressure over the internal ring when patient asked to cough. If hand is then removed, **impulse passes medially towards external ring and is palpable above the pubic tubercle**.

Direct inguinal hernia: impulse in a forward direction mainly above groin crease **above the pubic tubercle** and swelling not controlled by pressure over internal ring.

In fact it is very difficult to differentiate a direct from indirect inguinal hernia by examination alone. Even experienced surgeons are only correct 50% of the time. It is more important at the time of surgery and clinically mainly important to differentiate inguinal from femoral herniae. Femoral herniae are more likely to become irreducible and obstruct than inguinal as they usually have a smaller defect to protrude from.

Femoral hernia: swelling fills out the groin crease medial to the femoral artery, and more importantly below the pubic tubercle.

Examination of genitals

- **Ask in a sensitive way** before you proceed, e.g. 'I should briefly examine you down below. Is that all right?'
- **In the male, palpate the scrotum** for the testes and epididymes. It is rarely necessary to examine the penis.

Tender and enlarged testes may occur with *orchitis* or *torsion of the testis*.

A **large, hard, painless testis** suggests *cancer*.

A **large, soft swelling which transilluminates** suggests *hydrocele* or an *epididymal cyst*. A hydrocele surrounds the testis; an epididymal cyst lies behind the testis.

Balanitis (inflamed glans of penis) should remind the examiner to check for diabetes.

Per rectum examination

Never perform a rectal examination without permission from the F1 doctor or registrar or without a chaperone. Most medical schools use prosthetic training models for this examination to be practised prior to examining patients.

- Tell the patient at each stage what you are going to do.
- Lie the patient on the left side with knees flexed to the chest.
- Say: 'I am going to put a finger into your back passage'.
- Inspect anus for haemorrhoids and fissures.
- With lubricant on glove, gently insert forefinger into rectum. Feel the tone of the sphincter, size and character of the prostate and any lateral masses. If appropriate, proceed to proctoscopy.
- Test stool on your glove for occult blood. Then clean the patient's perineum with a tissue and wash your hands after disposing of the glove.

Per vaginam examination

Never perform a vaginal examination without a chaperone, female if possible, and only on the direction of a qualified instructor.

- Tell the patient at each stage what you are going to do.
- Lie the patient on her back with hips flexed and abducted (although some physicians prefer the patient lying on her left side as for per rectum examination).
- Inspect the external genitalia.
- With lubricant on glove insert one finger into vagina and then a second finger if there is room.
- Palpate the cervix.
- Examine for position and enlargement of uterus, tenderness of appendages and masses.
- Check for discharge by observing glove. Then offer the patient a tissue and wash your hands after disposing of the gloves.

Summary of common illnesses

Cirrhosis

- white nails
- clubbing
- liver palms
- spider naevi
- jaundice
- firm liver

Portal hypertension

- splenomegaly
- ascites
- caput medusa

Hepatic encephalopathy

- liver flap
- drowsy
- constructional apraxia (cannot draw five-pointed star)
- musty foetor

'Dehydration' (water and salt loss)

- dry skin
- veins collapsed
- diminished skin turgor—pinched fold of skin remains raised
- tongue dry
- eyes sunken
- blood pressure low with postural drop

Intestinal obstruction

- patient 'dehydrated' if they have been vomiting
- abdomen centrally swelling
- visible peristalsis
- not tender (unless inflammation, or some other pathology)
- resonant to percussion
- loud 'tinkling' bowel sounds

Pyloric stenosis

- upper abdomen swelling
- may have 'succussion splash' on shaking abdomen
- otherwise like intestinal obstruction

Appendicitis

- slight fever
- deep tenderness of right iliac fossa over McBurney's point (or rarely per rectum)

- otherwise little to find unless has spread to peritonitis

Peritonitis
- lies still
- abdomen
  - does not move on respiration
  - rigid on palpation (guarding)
  - tender, particularly on removing fingers rapidly (rebound tenderness)
- absent bowel sounds

Cholecystitis
- tender right hypochondrium, particularly on breathing in (Murphy's sign—tender gallbladder descends on inspiration to touch your palpating hand)

Jaundice and palpable gallbladder
- obstruction is not due to gallstones, but from another obstruction such as a neoplasm of the pancreas (Courvoisier's law). Gallstones have usually caused a fibrosed gallbladder, which cannot dilate from back-pressure from gallstones in common bile duct

Enlarged spleen
- infective, e.g. *septicaemia* or *subacute bacterial endocarditis*
- portal hypertension, e.g. *cirrhosis*
- *lymphoma*, leukaemia and other haematological diseases
- autoimmune, e.g. systemic lupus, Felty's syndrome

System-oriented examination

'Examine the abdomen'
- hands: clubbing, liver flap, Dupuytren's contracture
- eyes: jaundice, anaemia
- tongue: foetor, smooth

- neck: Virchow's lymph node
- chest: spider naevi, gynaecomastia
- palpate inguinal lymph nodes briefly
- inspect abdomen asymmetry, movement, pulsation, swelling
- enquire whether pain or tenderness
- palpate all nine areas of the abdomen for masses: note abdominal tenderness, guarding, rigidity
- palpate liver, kidneys, spleen, aortic aneurysm
- ascites: test for shifting dullness
- auscultate bowel sounds, arterial or liver bruits
- examine for hernia: ask patient to cough. Stand patient up if a hernia is a possibility
- enquire whether appropriate:
  - to examine vulva/testes/scrotum
  - to do rectal examination

CHAPTER 6

Examination of the mental state

Introduction

Examination of the mental state is necessary in all patients, not just those seen in psychiatric settings. The main headings are:

- **appearance and behaviour**
- **mood**
- **speech**—rate, form, content
- **thinking**—form, content
- **abnormal beliefs**—odd ideas and delusions
- **abnormal perceptions**—hallucinations and illusions
- **cognitive function**—concentration, orientation, memory, reasoning
- **understanding of condition**.

The distinction between history and examination becomes blurred when examining disordered mental states.

Much of the examination is done by careful observation while taking the history, and then supplemented with additional questions afterwards (see Chapter 1 under Mental state and Chapter 7 under Cognitive function).

If there is difficulty obtaining a clear history or if the patient appears distressed, it is particularly important to examine the mental state.

General rules

- Be non-judgemental.
- Be alert to phenomena that are observed.

Clinical Skills and Examination: The Core Curriculum. By R Turner, B Angus, A Handa, C Hatton. ©2009 Blackwell Publishing, ISBN: 9781405157513.

- Do not jump to conclusions about what the patient is saying.
- Clarify with gentle enquiry:
  - **'Can you tell me more about that?'**
  - **'Can you give me a recent example?'**
  - **'When did that last happen?'**
  - **'What did you do about it?'**
  - **'How often/how long have you experienced that?'**

Appearance and behaviour (observation)

- Describe in simple terms:
  - unkempt appearance
  - bewildered, agitated, restless, aggressive, tearful, sullen:
    - appropriate to setting?
    - reduced activity in *depression*
    - overactive and intrusive in *mania*
    - tense and reassurance seeking with *anxiety*
  - able to respond to questions
  - evidence of responding to hallucinations
  - smell of alcohol
  - evidence of drug misuse (e.g. needle marks).

Mood (part observation, part enquiry)

Mood is a subjective state and is mainly judged by the impression conveyed during the history, although examination gives further clues.

- Ask:
  - **'How have your spirits been recently?'**
  - **'Have you been feeling your normal self?'**
  - **'Is this how you normally feel?'**

Depressed—depression disorder or an adjustment reaction (see questions following).

Elevated—manic disorder or intoxication, e.g. ethanol, drugs, delirium.

Anxious—anxiety disorder or reaction to situation.

Angry—delirium or reaction to situation.

Flat—depressed or no emotional rapport, i.e. *schizophrenia*.

- If evidence for depression, worry, agitation, irritability—record current nature and severity.
  - If depressed, ask:
    - 'How bad has it been?'
    - 'Have you ever thought of suicide?'
    - 'Have you seriously considered taking your life?'
- Also ask for nurses' and relatives' comments.

Speech (observation)

Describe speech in simple terms and record verbatim typical remarks.

- **Rate:**
  - fast in *mania*
  - slow in *depression*.
- **Form:**
  - are there abnormalities of grammar or flow? Record examples

Disordered thought processes can occur in *schizophrenia, mania, acute organic states, dementia*.

  - are there abnormal sequences of words?
    - non sequiturs with disordered logic in *schizophrenia*—'word jumble'
    - loosely connected topics in *mania*—'flight of ideas'.
- **Content** (observations, elaborate with enquiry):
  - 'You said you . . . , tell me more about that'
  - 'When you feel sad, what goes through your mind?'

Thinking (form and content—largely inferred from speech)

- Record patient's main thoughts or preoccupations:
  - negative pessimistic in *depression*—ask about suicidal intentions
  - grandiose in *mania*
  - catastrophising in *anxiety*

Obsessions—intrusive thoughts or repetitious behaviours which the patient cannot resist although they know they are not sensible.

- perseveration—repetition of a word or phrase. Can occur in *anxiety, depression, mania, delirium* or *dementia*.

Abnormal beliefs (odd ideas and delusions)

- Ask to describe; be non-judgemental.
- Ask why they think that—may reveal psychotic thoughts or hallucinations.

Delusions are fixed, false beliefs without reasonable evidence, e.g. I've got AIDS/cancer.

- 'Did it ever seem to you that people were talking about you?'
- 'Have you ever received special messages from the television, radio or newspaper?'
- 'Do people seem to be going out of their way to get at you?'
- 'Have you ever felt that you were especially important in some way or that you had special powers?'
- 'Do you ever feel you have committed a crime or done something terrible for which you should be punished?'

Abnormal perceptions (hallucinations and illusions—usually apparent from history)

- Ask—'Have you had any unusual experiences recently?'
  - 'Do they seem as if they are in the real world or as if they are "inside" your head?'

Hallucinations are false perceptions without a stimulus (e.g. pink elephants—experienced as real).

- They can occur in any sensory modality.
- Visual hallucinations are suggestive of an organic state.
- Third person ('he' or 'she') auditory hallucinations are suggestive of *schizophrenia*.
  - 'Do you ever hear things that other people can't hear, such as the voices of people talking?'
  - 'Do you ever have visions or see things that other people can't see?'
  - 'Do you ever have strange sensations in your body or skin?'

Illusions are misinterpreted perceptions (e.g. he thinks you are a policeman). They are common in acute organic states (*psychosis*).

Cognitive functioning (observations supplemented by specific enquiry)

- **Impairment of concentration** can occur in:
  - *depression*
  - *anxiety states*
  - *dementia*
  - *confusional state*.
- **Orientation, thought processes, memory and logic.** These aspects must be tested as part of examination of the mental state (see Chapter 7 under Cognitive function).

Understanding of condition

- **'What do you think is wrong with you?'**
  - **'Is there any illness that you are particularly worried about?'**
  - **'What treatment do you feel is appropriate?'**
  - **'Are there any treatments you are frightened of?'**

It is important to ask all patients these questions. If the patient lacks insight into abnormal beliefs or behaviour, this suggests a psychotic illness.

General history and examination

Mental illness can be the presentation of a physical illness and a full history and examination should be done in all patients.

Physical illnesses that masquerade as mental illnesses include:

- *infection especially urinary tract but also consider meningitis and encephalitis*
- *hypothyroid, hyperthyroid*
- *hypercalcaemia, hypokalaemia, hypomagnesaemia or hyponatraemia*
- *cerebral tumour*
- *other causes of increased intracranial pressure*

- *drugs*
- *porphyria.*

It is arguable that all mental illness arises from a physical imbalance of transmitters/receptor function in the brain, and the division of illness into physical and mental is spurious. In any case, all patients, whatever the nature of their illness, should be treated non-judgementally and with respect.

Problem patients

Angry patients

- Inordinate anger is often symptomatic of another problem.
- Assess whether the grievance is justified and whether it can be resolved.
- 'Is there anything else that is upsetting you?'
- If the antagonism is directed against you, enquire whether the patient would prefer to see somebody else.

Aggressive patients

- Do not take risks (have help nearby and do not let the patient sit between you and the door).
- Ensure the patient does not have a weapon.
- Determine orientation and whether the patient is intoxicated or deluded.
- Fear often underlines aggression—what is the fear?

Tearful patients

- If a patient starts to weep, be calm and gently sympathetic.
- When less tearful, enquire why they are upset. If you can find out the reason:
  - it may help rapport
  - it may allow resolution of the problem.

Suicidal patients

- Assess intent of recent attempt (if any):
  - planning and likelihood of discovery
  - perceived dangerousness of method
  - intention at the time.

- Assess current intent:
  - how likely is the patient to attempt suicide?
  - what do they want to happen?
  - what would increase/decrease the risk?

Embarrassed patients

- Patients may not wish to talk about a distressing situation.
- It may help to reassure about confidentiality.
- If you think you know the problem, you can bring it up:
  - 'Is there a problem with money/sex/children, etc?'
- If the patient really does not want to talk about a problem, it is better to leave it and broach it later, possibly at another interview. Women may wish to discuss with a female doctor or student.

Talkative patients

Some patients go into irrelevant detail, digress and repeat themselves.

- Remind the patient of the time left and need to cover main points. Check what they are and proceed.
- Politely say, 'Thank you. Please help me with some specific questions . . .' and proceed to specific questions that require answers.

Nonsense history

- Occasionally you get nowhere—contradictory remarks, description of improbable events, perseveration or just silence and monosyllables.
- Change to other aspects of history, e.g. personal or family history, social circumstances.
- If these also do not help, proceed if feasible to examination. You may identify *dementia, evidence of drug abuse, hysteria* or some other illness that explains the problem.
- Essential to interview other informants (e.g. telephone a relative).

Summary of common illnesses

Depression

- low mood, tearfulness (not always present)
- lack of interest and self-care
- poor concentration
- negative thought content
- low self-esteem
- wakes up early
- depressed facies
- slow movements and speech
- weight loss
- negative speech content

Anxiety

- generally worried
- thought focuses on catastrophes
- cannot get to sleep
- tense, lined face, furrowed brow
- sweaty palms
- shaky
- hyperventilation
- tachycardia

Anorexia nervosa

- thin, little body fat
- increased, fine body hair
- sees self as fat even if thin
- thoughts dominated by food

Bulimia nervosa

- often normal weight
- binges followed by self-induced vomiting
- thoughts dominated by food
- erosion of teeth from vomiting

Acute psychosis *(schizophrenia, mania or depressive psychosis)*

- alert and oriented
- normal activities disrupted

- unpredictable behaviour
- reports or behaves as if responding to hallucinations
- reports delusional beliefs

Schizophrenic psychosis
- illogical thought, even a disjointed 'word salad'
- auditory hallucinations (third person)
- delusions (especially concerning thoughts, e.g. broadcast)
- activity may be responding to hallucinations and delusions

Manic psychosis
- rapid speech with 'flight of ideas'
- overactive, cannot keep still
- normal activities disrupted
- overly cheerful or irritable
- stands close and is argumentative

Depressive psychosis
- depressed affect
- slow movements and speech
- negative thoughts and delusions, e.g. brain is rotting
- suicidal thoughts

Chronic schizophrenia
- alert and oriented
- unkempt
- odd, rambling speech
- elaborate delusions
- mannerisms and odd gestures
- look for tardive dyskinesia (parkinsonian features from long-term neuroleptic treatment)

Delirium
- fluctuating level of concentration and orientation—worse at night
- fleeting delusions, often persecutory in nature
- evidence of toxicity (fever, etc.)

Intoxication (a type of delirium)

- smells of alcohol or glue
- needle marks
- impaired alertness and drowsy
- visual hallucinations

Dementia

- alert (unless also delirious)
- may be unkempt
- poor orientation in time and space
- cognitive function subnormal
  - poor short-term memory
  - cannot remember recent events
  - cannot remember and repeat series of numbers or an address
  - cannot explain proverbs
- paucity of thought and speech

Bereavement

- low mood and tearfulness when thinking of lost person
- may have somatic symptoms
- assess suicide risk (to join lost person)
- if excessively severe or prolonged (more than 6 months), may be considered 'pathological'

Somatisation/hypochondriasis

- somatic symptoms (often pain, fatigue) with no organic disease
- assess for sign of depression
- determine patient's illness, fears or beliefs
- symptoms are main concern in *somatisation*, fear of illness in *hypochondriasis*

CHAPTER 7
Examination of the nervous system

Introduction

The goal of the examination is to answer three questions:

1 Does the patient have a neurological illness?
2 Where in the nervous system is the pathology located?
3 What is the pathology?

As always, the history is critical. The following features in the history can be informative:

- **onset**
  - abrupt—*vascular, mechanical*
  - seconds—*seizure*
  - minutes—*migraine*
  - hours—*infective, inflammatory*
  - days/weeks—*neoplasm* or *degenerative disorder*
- **duration**
  - brief episodes with recovery, e.g. *TIA, epilepsy, migraine, syncope*
  - longer episodes with recovery—*mechanical, obstruction* or *pressure*
  - demyelination, e.g. *multiple sclerosis*
- **frequency**
- **witness description**—particularly if the patient has episodic loss of consciousness or is confused.

The examination of the nervous system can be elaborated almost indefinitely. Of far greater importance is **to acquire the ability to conduct a thorough but**

Clinical Skills and Examination: The Core Curriculum. By R Turner, B Angus, A Handa, C Hatton. ©2009 Blackwell Publishing, ISBN: 9781405157513.

comparatively rapid examination with confidence in the findings. It is best to develop your own basic system for doing the examination and to perform it consistently. This will avoid omissions.

- **Adapt your examination to the situation.** The routine examination must be mastered but can be altered to fit the situation.

The examination of the nervous system is approached under the following headings:

- **Higher cerebral function**
- **Cranial nerves**
- **Motor**
- **Coordination**
- **Reflexes**
- **Sensation**
- **Gait and station**

The nervous system cannot be examined in isolation. Other points of relevance may include:

- configuration of the skull and spine
- neck stiffness
- ear drums for otitis media
- blood pressure
- heart, e.g. arrhythmia, mitral stenosis
- carotid arteries—palpation and bruit
- neoplasms—breast, lung, abdominal
- jaundice.

Higher cerebral functions

Higher mental functions can only be properly assessed in an alert, awake and cooperative patient. From the history it is usually obvious whether it is necessary to examine the higher cerebral functions in detail. The ability to give a coherent history suggests normal higher mental function. A patient with sciatica would rightly be dismayed by an examination beginning with asking the patient to name the parts of a watch. However, if the patient is unable to give a coherent history, then cognitive testing is necessary.

General observation

- **Appearance**, e.g. unkempt.
- **Behaviour**, e.g. bewildered, restless, agitated.
- **Emotional state**, e.g. depressed, euphoric, hostile.

Observe, and ask for nurses' and relatives' comments.

Conscious level

If the patient is not fully conscious shake them gently or speak to them loudly.

The Glasgow Coma Scale

The GCS provides a rapid, widely used assessment of level of consciousness. Monitor responses to verbal command or, if no response, to painful stimulus, e.g. supraorbital pressure (with thumb nail in supraorbital groove), sternal rub (with knuckles over ribs), nailbed pressure (with thumb nail), twist fold of skin (but do not leave a bruise). It is helpful to record a description of the patient as well as the GCS score (out of 15).

Add up the total from A, B, C below.

	Score	
A Eye opening	1	Eyes remain closed
	2	Eyes open to pain
	3	Eyes open to command
	4	Spontaneous with normal blinking
B Verbal response	1	No response
	2	Incomprehensible, moaning sounds only
	3	Inappropriate—words spoken but no conversation
	4	Confused speech
	5	Normal speech
C Motor response	1	No response
	2	Extensor reflex response to pain—adduction and internal rotation at shoulder, extension at elbows, pronation of forearms

C Motor response (continued)	3 Flexor reflex response to pain—withdrawal of limb
	4 Withdrawal of limb in response to pain
	5 Localising: attempts to protect site of pain
	6 Voluntary: responds normally to commands

Confusion

If a patient appears confused, move on to assess cognitive state, including disorientation (see under Cognitive function). Make sure the patient does not have a receptive aphasia first (see below).

Language/speech

Assess from conversation.

- **Is there difficulty in articulation?** If necessary, ask patient to say 'British Constitution', 'West Register Street'.
  - **Dysarthria**
    - cerebellar—scanning or staccato
    - lower motor neuron
    - palatal palsy—nasal
    - upper motor neuron—slow, 'spastic', seen in pseudobulbar palsy
    - acute alcohol poisoning.
- **Is there altered voice tone?**
    - extrapyramidal (monotonous and slow).
  - **Dysphonia**
    - cord lesion—hoarse
    - hysterical.
- **Is there difficulty in finding the right word?**
  - **Dysphasia** or **aphasia**—disorder of use of words as symbols in speech, writing and understanding. Nearly always due to left hemiphere lesion.

  N.B. Right- or left-handed? May be right hemisphere lesion if left-handed.
  - **Expressive dysphasia**—difficulty finding words; speech slow and hesitant, may use circumlocutions;

due to a lesion in Broca's area. Test for by asking patient to name objects you point to, e.g. wristwatch, pen, tie. Comprehension should be intact.

- **Receptive dysphasia**—speech fluent, but comprehension poor; patient may seem 'confused'. Test for by asking patient to follow commands—a three-step command is a good screening test (e.g. 'please pick up the glass, but first point to the curtain and then the door'). Due to a lesion in Wernicke's area.
- **Mixed dysphasia**—most common; spontaneous speech scanty, small vocabulary, often with wrong words used, comprehension impaired. There are also other dysphasias produced by interruption of the connecting pathways between the speech centres.
- **Mutism**—no speech at all. This may be due to aphasia, anarthria, psychiatric disease or, occasionally, diffuse cerebral pathology.

Other defects occurring in the absence of motor or sensory dysfunction

- **Dyslexia**—inappropriate difficulty with reading. Read few lines from newspaper (having established that comprehension and expressive speech are intact).
- **Dysgraphia**—loss of ability to write.
- **Acalculia**—loss of ability to do mental and written sums.
- **Apraxia**—inability to perform a purposeful task when no motor or sensory loss, e.g. opening matchbox, waving goodbye. Apraxia for dressing is common in *diffuse brain disease*. Inability to draw five-pointed star occurs in *hepatic pre-coma*.
- **Agnosia**—inability to recognise objects (e.g. a key or coin when placed in hand. Tactile agnosia = **astereognosis**).
- **Parietal lobe lesions**—especially right, cause spatial difficulties; getting lost in familiar places, inability to

lay table or draw or make patterns with matches, neglect of left side of space, or of half of body.

Cognitive function

Take account of any evidence you have about the patient's intelligence, education and interests.

'Cognitive' is a term that covers **orientation**, **thought processes and logic**. **Regular use of a simple mental state test is suggested.** The section below describes some aspects of cognitive testing in more detail.

Orientation

- **Check awareness of:**
  - **time**: 'What day is it?' (time, month, year)
  - **place**: 'Where are you?'
  - **person**: 'What is your name?'

Disorientation suggests *acute organic state* or *dementia*. *Depressed patients* may be unwilling to reply although they know the answers.

Attention and calculation

- Tests of concentration include asking the patient to take away 7 from 100, 7 from 93, etc.; 20 minus 3 in another simpler version of this test; or by asking for the months of the year backwards, or by spelling the word 'world' backwards.

Concentration may be impaired with many *cerebral abnormalities especially delirium*, *depression* and *anxiety*.

Memory

Immediate recall—digit span

- Repeat digits spoken slowly. Start with an easy short sequence and then increase the numbers. Most people manage seven digits forwards, five backwards.

Short-term memory

- **Ask patient to tell you:**
  - what they had for breakfast
  - what they did the night before

- what they have read in today's paper
- recent topical news items. This should be geared to the patient's interests, e.g. football results for an avid football fan.

Demented patients will be unable to do this. They may **confabulate** (make up impressive stories) to cover their ignorance (particularly likely in alcohol-related dementia).

New memory

- Give a name and address, make sure the patient has learnt it, and then test recall at 5 minutes.

Longer-term memory

- Ask patient:
  - for events before illness, e.g. last year, or during last week
  - 'What is your address?'

General knowledge

- Assess in relation to anticipated performance from history.
  - what is the name of the Queen/President/Prime Minister?
  - name six capital cities
  - what were the dates of the last war?

In *acute organic states* and *dementia*, new learning, recent memory and reasoning appear to be more impaired than remote memory. Vocabulary is usually well-preserved in *dementia*. In *depression*, patients may be unwilling to reply, and appear demented.

  - a history from a relative or employer is very important in early dementia, particularly for ability to function. Demented patients tend not to be able to work appropriately or drive safely; anxious and depressed patients usually can.

Reasoning (abstract thought)

- What would you do if you found a stamped addressed envelope on the ground?

Skull and spine

- **Inspect and palpate skull** if there is any possibility of a head injury.
- **Check neck stiffness**—meningeal irritation (see under Signs of meningeal irritation)
- **Inspect spine**—usually when examining back of chest.
- If there is any possibility of pathology, stand the patient and check all movements of the spine.

Cranial nerves

Examine cranial nerves and upper limbs with the patient sitting up, preferably on the side of the bed or on a chair.

I Olfactory

Not normally tested. Occasionally can be useful if there are other neurological defects, including papilloedema, undiagnosed headache or head injury. Ask if there has been a change in the sense of smell.

Oil of cloves, peppermint, coffee, etc.—each nostril in turn. It is normal not to be able to name smells, but one smell should be distinguished from another.

Pungent or noxious smells such as ammonia should not be used.

Abnormal:

- *rhinitis*
- *head injury*
- *olfactory groove meningioma*
- *smoking.*

II Optic

Visual acuity

- **Test each eye separately. Ask if the patient normally wears glasses for distance or reading and ask them to wear them as appropriate.**
- **Ask the patient to read small newspaper print** with each eye separately, **with reading glasses if used. If sight is poor, test formally:**
  - **near vision**—newsprint or **Jaeger type** (each eye in

turn) (see Appendix 1)
- **distant vision—Snellen type** (more precise method) (see Appendix 2).

Stand patient at 6 m from Snellen's card (each eye in turn). Results expressed as a ratio:
- 6—distance of person from card
- *x*—distance at which the patient should be able to read type

i.e. 6/6 is good vision, 6/60 means the smallest type the patient can read is large enough to be normally read at 60 m.

If the patient cannot read 6/6, try after correction with glasses or pinhole. Looking through a pinhole in a card obviates refractive errors, analogous to a pinhole camera. If vision remains poor, suspect a neurological or ophthalmic cause.

A 3 m Snellen chart is shown in Appendix 2.

A pinhole is not effective for correcting near vision for reading.

Visual fields

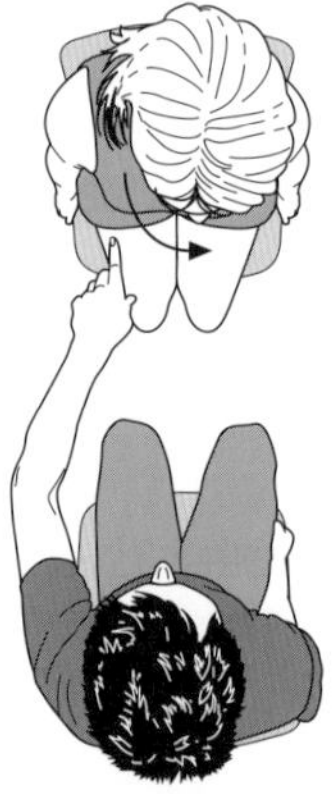

- Quick method for **temporal peripheral fields** by confrontation of the patient and examiner with both eyes open. Always test fields—patients are often unaware of visual loss, the most dramatic of which is Anton's syndrome (blindness with lack of awareness of the blindness).
  - Sit opposite and ask the patient to look at your nose.
  - Examine each eye in turn.
  - Bring waggling finger forwards from behind the patient's ear in upper and lower lateral quadrants and ask when it can be seen.
    - Normal vision is approximately 100° from axis of eye.

The patient must fully understand the test. The extreme of peripheral vision can be tested with both eyes open, since the nose obstructs vision from the other eye. **If peripheral field appears restricted**, re-test with other eye covered to ensure each eye is being tested separately.

- Quick method for **nasal peripheral fields** by confrontation of patient and examiner with the other eye covered.
  - Normal vision is approximately 50° from each axis of eye.
- **Standard method.** With a small red pinhead held in the plane midway between the patient and examiner. With the other eye covered, compare the visual fields of patient with that of examiner, with the pin brought in from temporal or nasal fields.

  Defects in the central field can be assessed by the standard method with a small red pin held in the plane midway between the patient and examiner:
  - **scotoma**—defects in the central field (*retinal or optic nerve lesion*)
  - **enlarged blind spot** (*papilloedema*).

  Map by moving pen from inside scotoma or blind spot outwards until red pinhead reappears.

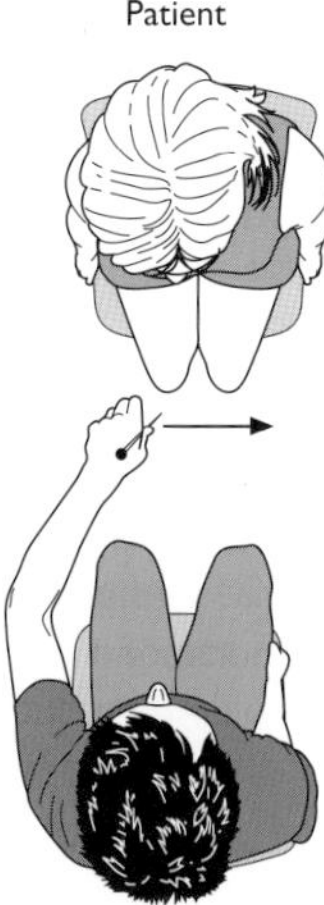

This is a crude test and small areas of loss of vision may need to be formally tested with a **perimetry**.

- **Test for sensory inattention** when fields are full with both eyes open.
  - Hold your hands between you and the patient, one opposite each ear and waggle forefingers simultaneously. Ask which moves. With a parietal defect, patient may not recognise

movement on one side, although fields are full to formal testing.

- **In a semiconscious patient a gross homonymous hemianopia** can be detected by a reflex blink to your hand rapidly passing by the eye towards the ear (menace reflex).
    - **Homonymous hemianopia** field defect (Figure 7.1), arising from lesions behind chiasma, is on same side as hemiparesis, if present.
    - **Top-quadrant defect**—from *temporal damage* or *occipital lesion*.

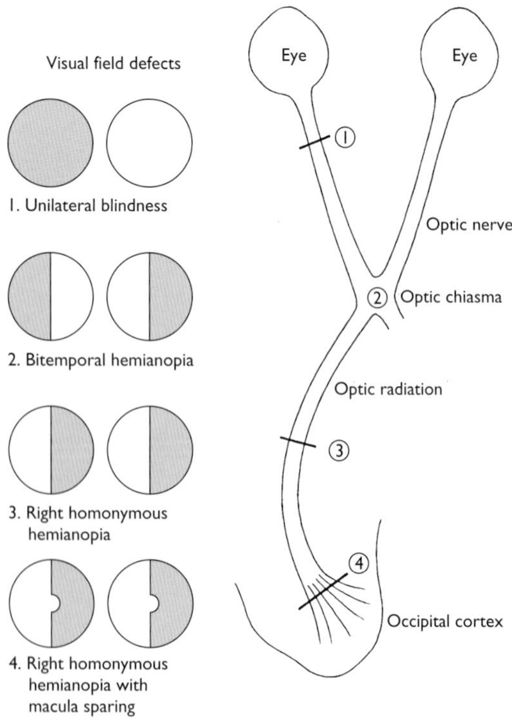

Figure 7.1 Visual field defects.

- **Lower-quadrant defect**—from *parietal damage* or *occipital lesion*.
- **Bitemporal defect**—from *pituitary lesion*.

Examine the fundi (see Chapter 2)

- Lesions particularly relevant to neurological system:
  - *optic atrophy*—pale disc and demyelination, e.g. *multiple sclerosis: pressure on nerve*
  - *papilloedema*—increased intracranial pressure:
    - *tumour*
    - *benign intracranial hypertension*
    - *hydrocephalus*
    - *non-communicating* (obstructed outflow via fourth ventricle)
    - *communicating*—block of cerebrospinal fluid uptake in spinal cord.
- A sensitive test for nystagmus is to ask the patient to cover the other eye during fundoscopy. This removes fixation and can help to elicit nystagmus.

II and III pupils

- **Look at pupils.** Are they round and equal?
  - **Symmetric small pupils:**
    - *old age*
    - *opiates*
    - *Argyll Robertson pupils (syphilis)* are small, irregular, eccentric pupils, reacting to convergence but not light
    - pilocarpine eye drops for narrow-angle glaucoma
    - iritis.
  - **Symmetric large pupils:**
    - *youth*
    - *alcohol*
    - *sympathomimetics, anxiety*
    - *atropine-like substances*.
  - **Asymmetric pupils:**
    - *third-nerve palsy*—affected pupil dilated, often with ptosis and diplopia
    - *Horner's syndrome* (sympathetic defect)—

affected pupil constricted, often with partial ptosis, enophthalmos and anhydrosis
   - *iris trauma*
   - *drugs* (see above).
- **Light reflex.** Shine bright light from a torch into each pupil in turn in a dimly lit room. Do pupils contract equally?
   - *Holmes–Adie pupil*: large, slowly reacting to light.
   - *Afferent defect, ocular or optic nerve blindness*: neither pupil responds to light in blind eye; both respond to light in normal eye.
   - Relative afferent defect
      - direct response appears normal but when light moves from normal to deficient eye, paradoxical dilation of pupil occurs
   - *Efferent defect—third-nerve lesion*, pupil does not respond to light in either eye.
- **Accommodation reflex.** Ask patient to look at distant object, and then at your finger 10–15 cm from nose—do pupils contract?
   - Response to accommodation but not light:
     Argyll Robertson
     Holmes–Adie
     occular blindness
     midbrain lesion
     some recovering *third-nerve lesions*.

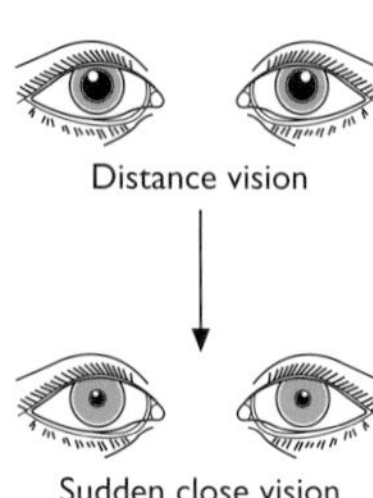

III Oculomotor

IV Trochlear

VI Abducens

External ocular movements

- **Test the eye movements in the four cardinal directions** (left, right, up, down) and convergence using your finger at 1 m distance. Look for abnormal eye movements.

- **Say: 'Tell me if you see double'.**

Upward gaze and convergence are often reduced in uncooperative patients.

- To detect minor lesions:
  - **Find direction of gaze with maximum separation of images.**
  - **Cover one eye and ask which image has gone.**

Peripheral image is seen by the eye that is not moving fully. **Peripheral image is displaced in direction of action of weak muscle**, e.g. maximum diplopia on gaze to left. Left eye sees peripheral image which is displaced laterally. Therefore left lateral rectus is weak.

Looking left

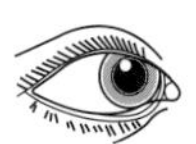
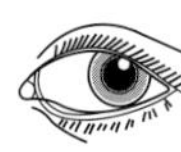

Normal

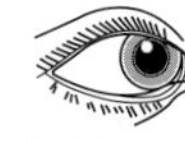
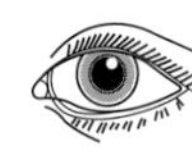

Left lateral rectus palsy (VI nerve)

Looking ahead

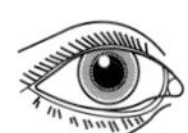
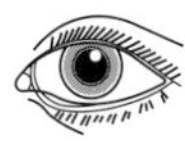

Normal

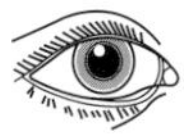
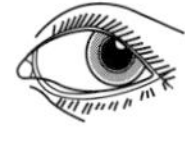

Left III nerve palsy

- **Diplopia** may be due to a single muscle or nerve lesion (N.B. monocular diplopia usually implies ocular pathology):
  - paralytic strabismus (squint)
    - **III palsy**: ptosis, large fixed pupil, eye can be abducted only; eye is often 'down and out'
    - **IV palsy**: diplopia when eye looks down or inwards
    - **VI palsy**: abduction paralysed, diplopia when looking to side of lesion (Figure 7.2)

- **concomitant non-paralytic strabismus**, e.g. *childhood ocular lesion*—constant angle between eyes. Usually no double vision as one eye ignored (amblyopic)

Looking right

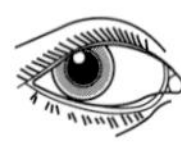
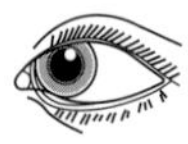
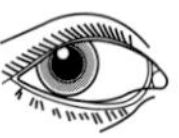
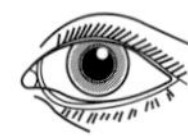

Looking ahead

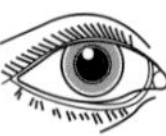
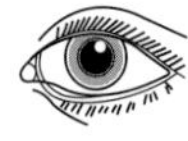
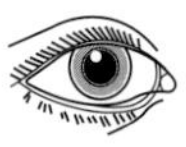
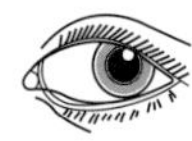

Normal

Concomitant strabismus with ambylopic left eye

- **conjugate ocular palsy**
  - *supranuclear palsies* affecting coordination rather than muscle weakness. Inability to look in particular direction, usually upwards
  - *intranuclear lesion*: convergence normal but cannot adduct eyes on lateral gaze

Looking ahead

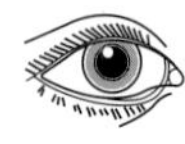
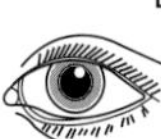
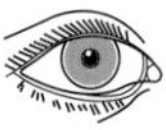
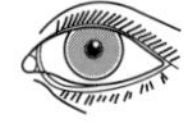

Looking up

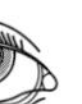
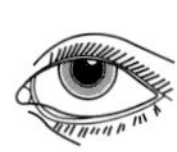
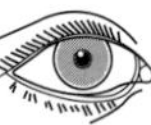
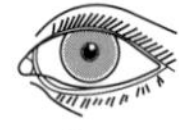

Normal

Supranuclear palsy

- if patient sees double in all directions
  - may be *third-nerve palsy*
  - *thyroid muscle disease*—worse in morning
  - myasthenia gravis—worse in evening
  - manifest strabismus.

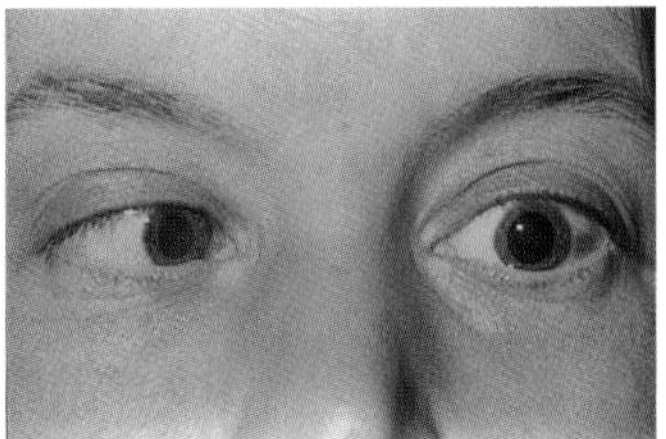

Figure 7.2 Left sixth nerve lesion—the patient is looking to the left, but there is no lateral movement of the left eye.

Ptosis

Drooping of upper eyelid can be:

- complete—*third-nerve palsy*
- incomplete
  - *partial third-nerve palsy*
  - fatigueable muscular weakness, e.g. *myasthenia gravis* (from anti-acetylcholine receptor antibodies)
  - sympathetic tone decreased—*Horner's syndrome* (also small pupils—enophthalmos and decreased sweating on face)
  - partial Horner's syndrome (small irregular pupils with ptosis) in *autonomic neuropathy of diabetes and syphilis*
  - lid swelling
  - levator dysinsertion syndrome (from chronic contact lens use).

Nystagmus

This is an unsteady eye movement. The flickering movement is labelled by the direction of fast movement.

- **Test first in the neutral position and then with the eyes deviated to right, left and upwards.** Keep object within binocular field as nystagmus is often normal in extremes of gaze.
  Characterised as primary when present with eyes at rest, or as gaze evoked, i.e. when produced by eye movement. Nystagmus is easier to detect with fixation removed. This can be done at the bedside during

ophthalmoscopy (see above). Remember, the nystagmus will appear in the opposite direction.

- **Cerebellar nystagmus**
  - fast movement to side of gaze (on both sides)
  - increased when looking to lesion
  - *cerebellar or brainstem lesion or drugs* (*ethanol, phenytoin*).

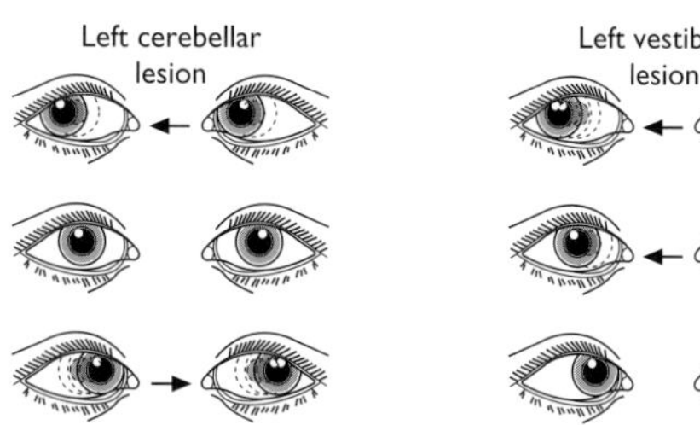

Fast phase looking to either side (see arrows) greater when looking to side of lesion. No nystagmus when looking ahead

Fast phase when looking away from lesion (see arrows); can also occur when looking ahead

- **Vestibular nystagmus**
  - fast movement only in one direction—away from lesion
  - reduced by fixation if peripheral in origin
  - more marked when looking away from lesion
    - *inner ear, vestibular disease or brainstem lesion*
    - labyrinthine nystagmus may be positional—particularly in benign positional vertigo, and can be induced by hyperextension and rotation of the neck (Hallpike manoeuvre) which after a latency of a few seconds will produce a vertical/torsional type of nystagmus for about 10–15 seconds, along with symptoms of vertigo.
- **Congenital nystagmus**—constant horizontal wobbling.
- Downbeat nystagmus—foramen magnum lesion or Wernicke's disease.
- Retraction nystagmus—midbrain lesion.

- Complex nystagmus—brainstem disease, usually multiple sclerosis.

Saccades

This is the rapid eye movement used to change eye position. It is tested in the horizontal and vertical planes, by asking the patient to switch fixation between two targets (e.g. the examiner's fingers). Slow saccades may be seen in a variety of disorders, including degenerative disorders such as progressive supranuclear palsy.

V Trigeminal

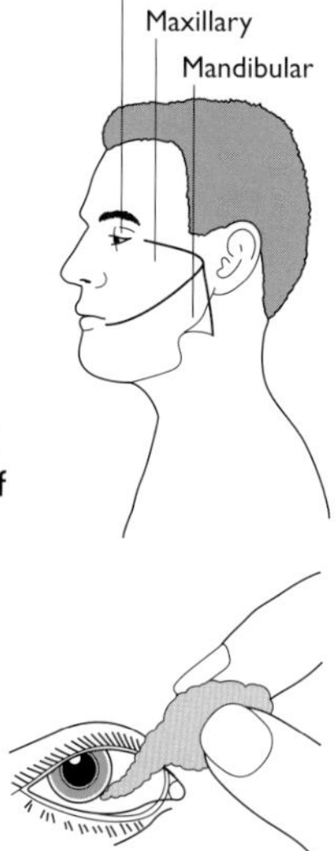

Sensory V

- **Test light touch in all three divisions.** A light touch with one's fingers is often adequate. Pinprick usually only if needed to delineate anaesthetic area.

Corneal reflex—sensory V and motor VII

- **Ask the patient to look up, and touch the cornea with a wisp of cotton wool.** Both eyes should blink. Remember the cornea is clear; do not test the sclera!

The corneal reflex is easily prompted incorrectly by eliciting the 'eyelash' or 'menace' reflex.

Motor V—muscles of jaw

- **Ask the patient to clench their teeth and feel the bulk of the masseter muscles for wasting.**
- **Ask the patient to open his mouth against resistance**, and look to see if jaw descends in midline. Palsy of the nerve causes deviation of the jaw to the side of the lesion.

Fifth-nerve palsies are very rare in isolation.

- **Jaw jerk**—only if other neurological findings, e.g. upper motor neuron lesion. Increased jaw jerk is only present if there is a bilateral upper motor neuron fifth-nerve lesion, e.g. *bilateral strokes* or *pseudobulbar palsy*.

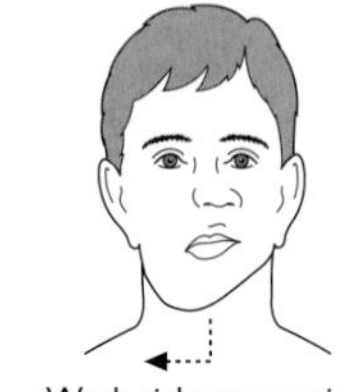

Weak right pterygoid

Put your forefinger gently on the patient's loosely opened jaw. Tap your finger gently with a tendon hammer. Explain the test to the patient or relaxation of his jaw will be impossible. A brisk jerk is a positive finding.

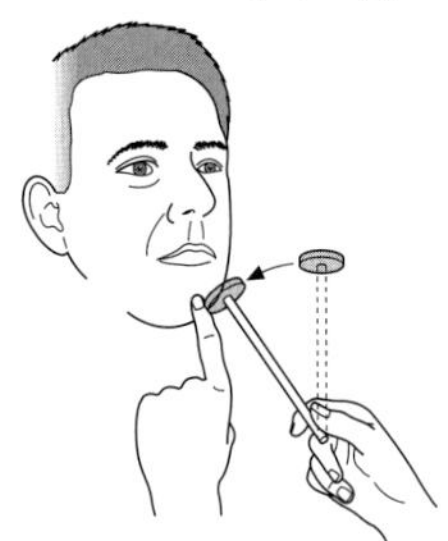

VII Facial

- **Ask the patient to:**
  - raise his eyebrows
  - close his eyes tightly
  - show you his teeth.

Demonstrate these to the patient yourself if necessary.

Lower motor neuron lesion: all muscles on the side of the lesion are affected, e.g. *Bell's palsy*: widened palpebral fissure, weak blink, drooped mouth.

Upper motor neuron lesion: only the lower muscles are affected, i.e. mouth drops to one side but eyebrows raise normally. This is because the part of the facial nucleus controlling the upper half of the face is bilaterally innervated. This abnormality is very common in a hemiparesis.

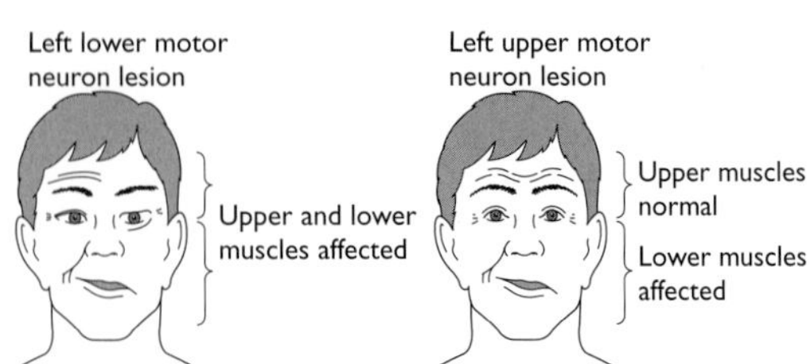

* **Taste** (chorda tympani): can only be tested easily on anterior two-thirds of the tongue.

VIII Auditory

Vestibular

No easy bedside test for this nerve except looking for nystagmus.

Acoustic

* **Block one ear by pressing the tragus. Whisper numbers increasingly loudly until the patient can repeat them.**

Rinne's test. Place a high-pitched vibrating tuning fork on the mastoid (1 in diagram). When the patient says the sound stops, hold the fork at the meatus (2 in diagram).

* If still heard: air conduction > bone conduction (normal or nerve deafness.
* If not heard: air conduction < bone conduction (middle-ear conduction defect).

Weber's test. Hold a vibrating tuning fork in the middle fot the patient's forehead. If sound is heard to one side, middle-ear deafness exists on that side or the opposing ear has nerve deafness.

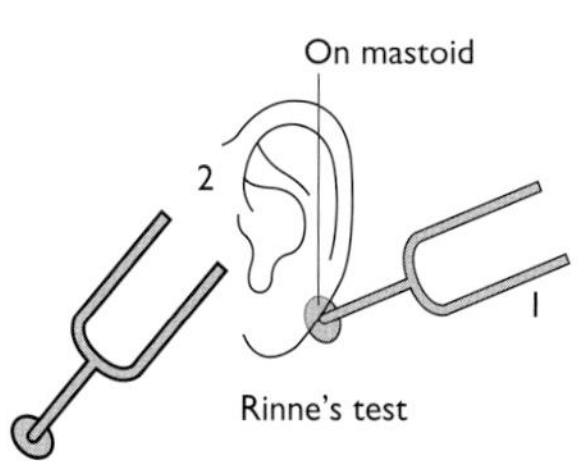

Rinne's test

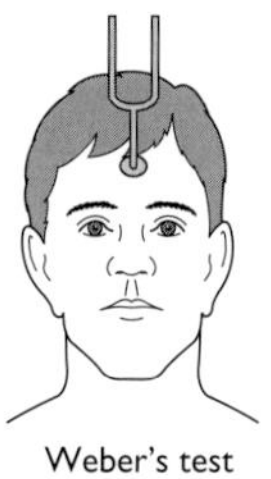
Weber's test

IX Glossopharyngeal

* **Ask patient to say 'Ahh'** and watch for symmetrical upwards movement of uvula—pulled away from weak side.
* **Gently touch the back of the pharynx with an orange stick** or spatula. If the patient gags the nerve is intact.

This gag reflex depends on the IX and X nerve, the former being the sensory side and the latter the motor aspect. It is frequently absent with ageing and abuse of tobacco.

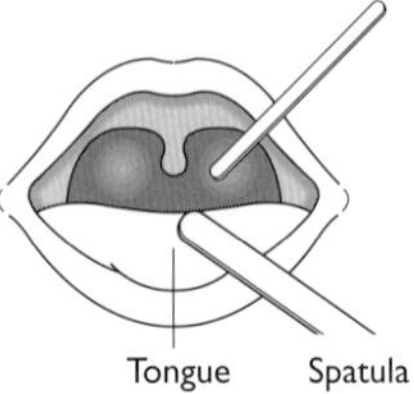

X Vagus

- **Ask if the patient can swallow normally.**

There are so many branches of the vagus nerve that it is impossible to be sure it is all functioning normally. If the vagus is seriously damaged, swallowing is a problem; spillage into the lungs may occur. Swallowing can be assessed by asking the patient to take a small drink of water. Observe the patient. Coughing on attempted swallow indicates a high risk of aspiration. Check speech afterwards—a change of voice quality ('wet' speech) indicates pooling of fluids on the vocal cords, and again indicates a high risk of aspiration. Check a voluntary cough—this can become quiet and ineffective.

- Check dysarthria (see under Language/speech).

XI Accessory

- **Ask the patient to flex neck**, pressing their chin against your resisting hand. Observe if both sternomastoids contract normally.
- **Ask the patient to raise both shoulders.** If they cannot, the trapezius muscle is not functioning.

Failure of the trapezius on one side is often associated with a *hemiplegia (particularly anterior cerebral artery infarctions)*. Traumatic cutting of the accessory nerve used to occur when tuberculous lymph glands of the neck were being excised.

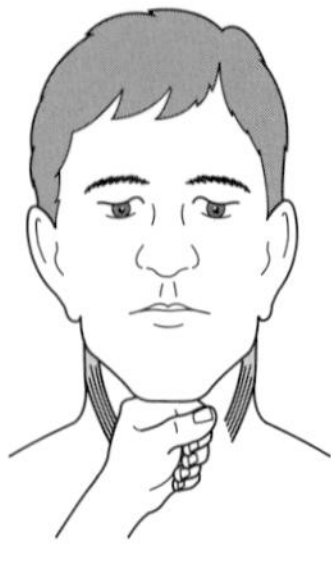

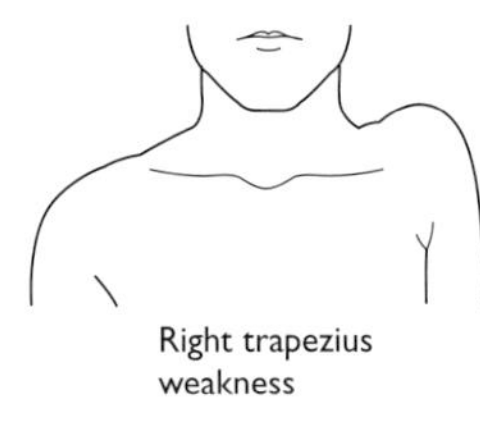

- **Ask the patient to turn the head against your resisting hand.** This tests the contralateral sternomastoid, and can help to demonstrate normal motor functioning in a hysterical hemiplegia.

XII Hypoglossal

- **Ask the patient to put out their tongue.** If it protrudes to one side, this is the side of the weakness, e.g. deviating to left on protrusion from left hypoglossal lesion.
- **Look for asymmetry, fasciculation or wasting** with mouth open.

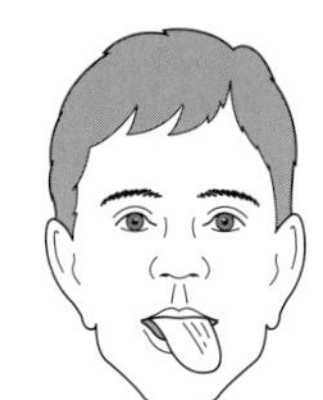

Left hypoglossal lesion

Limbs and trunk: motor, tone, coordination and reflexes

Remember the order of:

1. **Inspection**
2. **Tone**
3. **Power**
4. **Reflexes**
5. **Coordination**
6. **Sensation**

General inspection

- **Look at the patient's resting and standing posture:**
  - *hemiplegia*—flexed upper limb, extended lower limb
  - *wrist drop*—radial nerve palsy.
- **Look for abnormal movements:**
  - tremor
    - *Parkinson's*—coarse rhythmical tremor at rest, lessens on movement
    - essential tremor—tremor present on action; look at outstretched hands
    - *chorea*—abrupt, involuntary repetitive semi-purposeful movement
    - *athetosis*—slow, continuous writhing movement of limb.

- **Look for muscle wasting.** Check distribution:
  - symmetrical, e.g. *Duchenne muscular dystrophy*
  - asymmetrical, e.g. *poliomyelitis*
  - proximal, e.g. *limb-girdle muscular dystrophy*
  - distal, e.g. *peripheral neuropathy*
  - generalised, e.g. *motor neuron disease*
  - localised, e.g. with *joint disease*
- **Look for fasciculation.** This is irregular involuntary contractions of small bundles of muscle fibres.

  This is typical of denervation, e.g. *motor neuron disease when it is widespread*. It is caused by the death of anterior horn cells.

- **Ask the patient to hold both their arms straight out in front with the palms up and eyes shut.** Observe gross weakness, posture and whether arms remain stationary:
  - *hypotonic posture*—wrist flexed and fingers extended
  - *drift*—gradually upwards with sensory loss, especially parietal lobe
  - gradually downwards with pronation indicates *pyramidal weakness*
  - downward without pronation can be seen in hysteria or in profound proximal muscle weakness
  - athetoid tremors—sensory loss (peripheral nerve) or cerebellar disease
- **Tap both arms downwards.** They should reflexly return to their former position.

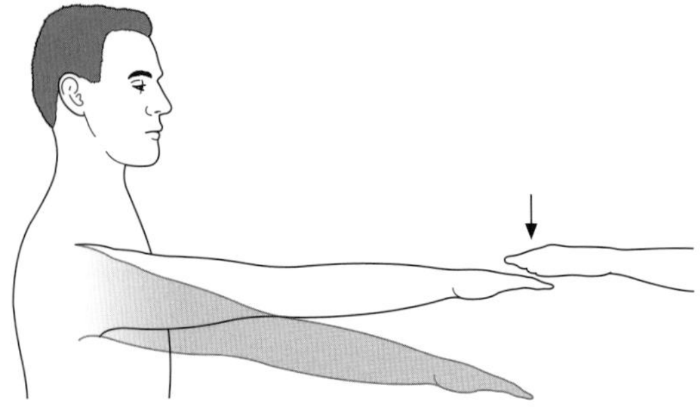

If the arm overswings in its return to its position, *weakness* or *cerebellar dysfunction* may be present.

- **Ask the patient to do fast finger movements**: 'Play a quick tune on the piano', demonstrating this yourself. Clumsy movements can be a sensitive index of a slight *pyramidal lesion*. The dominant side should always be quicker than the non-dominant.

Tone

Always check tone before you assess strength. This is a difficult test to perform as patients often do not relax. Try to distract the patient with conversation.

- **Ask the patient to relax their arm and then you flex and extend their wrist or elbow.** Move through a wide arc moderately slowly, at irregular intervals to prevent patient cooperation.
- **Ask the patient to let the limb go loose, lift it up and move at knee joint** (hip and ankle if required).

Difficult to assess in the legs because patients often cannot relax. Ankle clonus can be assessed at the same time (see below).

Hypertonia (increased tone):

- **pyramidal**: more obvious in flexion of upper limbs and extension of lower limbs. Occasionally 'clasp knife', i.e. diminution of tone during movement
- **extrapyramidal**: uniform 'lead pipe' rigidity. If associated with tremor the movement feels like a 'cog wheel'
- **hysterical**: increases with increased movement.

Hypotonia (decreased tone):

- *lower motor neuron lesion*
- recent *upper motor neuron lesion*
- *cerebellar lesion*
- *unconsciousness.*

Muscle power

- **For screening purposes, examine two distal muscles, one flexor and one extensor (e.g. finger flexion and extension), and two proximal muscles in each limb. Compare each side.** Confirm the weakness suspected by palpation of the muscle.

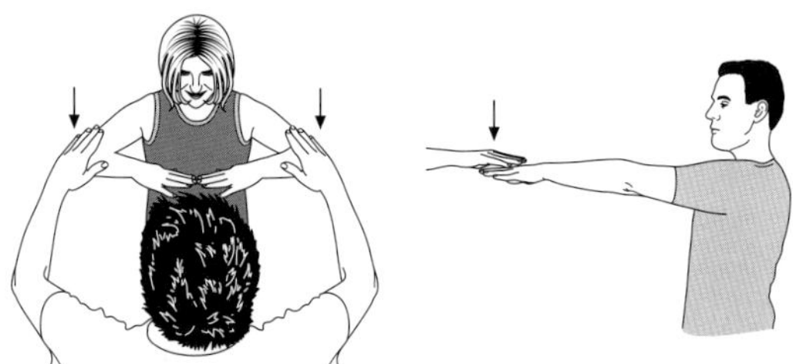

- If patient is in bed, start examination by asking them to:
  - raise both arms
  - raise one leg off the bed
  - raise the other leg off the bed.
- Test power at joints against your own strength—shoulder, elbow, wrist.

Power at main joints cannot normally be overcome by permissible force.

- **If there is weakness or other neurological signs in a limb, test individual muscle groups:**
  - shoulder—abduction, extension, flexion
  - elbow—flexion, extension
  - wrist—flexion, extension: 'Hold wrists up, don't let me push them down'
  - finger—flexion, grasp, extension, adduction (put a piece of paper between straight fingers held in extension and ask the patient to hold it, as you remove it), abduction (with fingers in extension, ask patient to spread them apart against your force)
- hip—flexion (ask patient to lift leg, 'don't let me push down') and extension (ask patient to keep

leg straight on bed, and try to lift at ankle); occasionally also abduction and adduction

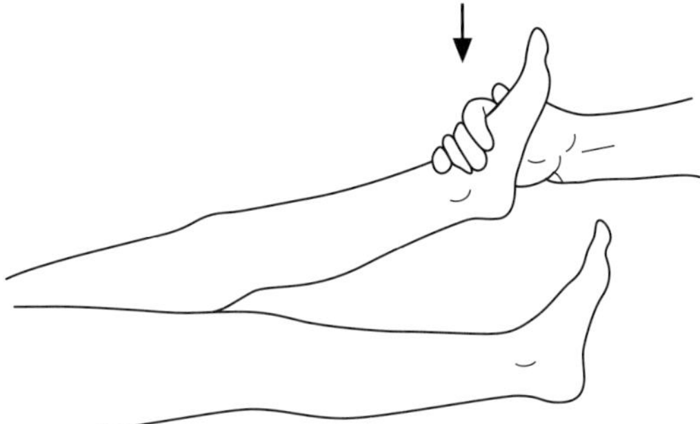

- knee—flexion, extension
- ankle—plantarflexion, dorsiflexion, eversion, inversion.

Only severe weakness will be detected because legs are stronger than arms. If no weakness is detected and patient is complaining of weakness, then more sensitive tests can be helpful, e.g. walking on tiptoes, heels, arising from a squat position, hopping on either leg.

Occasionally patients will have hysterical weakness. A useful test is Hoover's sign. This is tested by placing your hand under the ankle of the patient's paralysed leg. The patient is first asked to extend the paralysed leg (which should produce no effort). Then asking for hip flexion of the non-paralysed leg will result in contraction of the 'paralysed' hip extensor (a reflex fixation that we all do) if the weakness is hysterical. Unlike other tests for non-organic illness, this test demonstrates normalcy in the paralysed limb.

Strength is usually graded using the Medical Research Council scale as follows.

0 No active contraction.

1 Visible as palpable contraction with no active movement.

2 Movement with gravity eliminated, i.e. in horizontal direction.

3 Movement against gravity.

4 Movement against gravity plus resistance: it may be subdivided into 4– to 4+.

5 Normal power.

- Look for patterns of weakness:
  - *hemiplegia*—muscles weak all down one side
  - *monoplegia*—weakness of one limb
  - *paraplegia*—weakness of both lower limbs
  - *tetraplegia*—weakness of all four limbs
  - *myasthenia*—weakness developing after repeated contractions—most obvious in smaller muscles, e.g. repeated blinking (see under Ptosis)
  - proximal muscles, e.g. myopathy
  - nerve root distribution, e.g. disc prolapse
  - nerve distribution, e.g. wrist drop from radial nerve palsy.

Coordination

- **Ask the patient to touch their nose with their index finger.**
- **With the patient's eyes open, ask them to touch their nose, then your finger which is held up in front of them.** This can be repeated rapidly with your finger moving from place to place in front of him.

Missed!

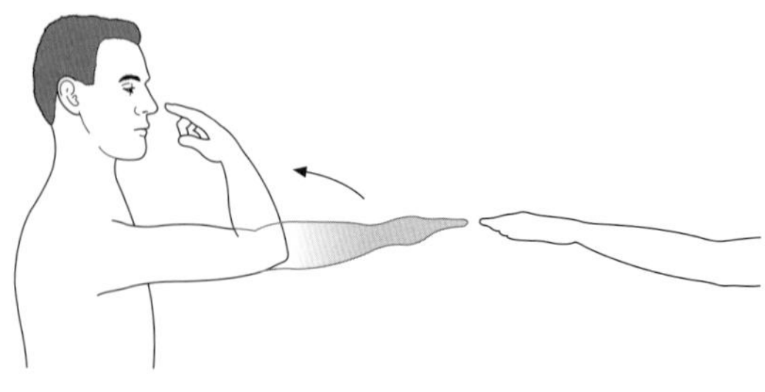

Past pointing and marked intention tremor in the absence of muscular weakness suggests *cerebellar dysfunction*. If you suspect a cerebellar abnormality check rapid alternating movements (*dysdiadochokinesia*):

- **fast rotation of the hands** (supination and pronation)
- **tapping back of other hand as quickly as possible.**

- Ask the patient to run the heel of one leg up and down the shin of the other leg. Lack of coordination will be apparent.
- Gait may become broad based, with the patient unable to perform a tandem gait (heel–toe walking).

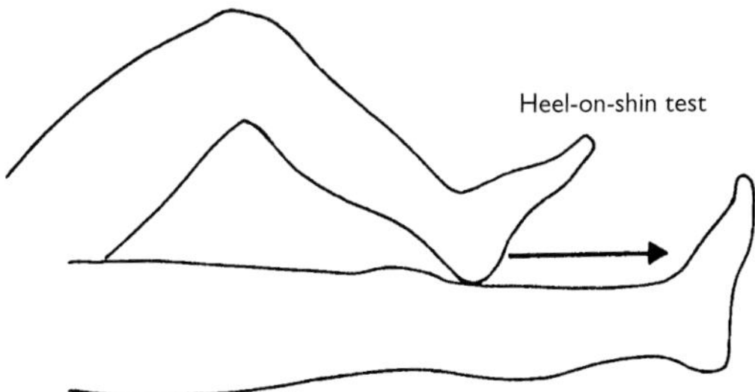

Tendon reflexes

- Place arms comfortably by the sides with elbows flexed and hand on upper abdomen. Tell the patient to relax.
- **Supinator reflex (root C5, C6):** tap the distal end of the radius with a tendon hammer.
- **Biceps reflex (root C5, C6):** tap your forefinger or thumb over biceps tendon.
- **Triceps reflex (root C7, C8):** hold arm across chest to tap the triceps tendon.
- **Knee reflexes (root L3, L4):** by passing left forearm behind both knees, supporting them partly flexed. Ask the patient to let their leg go loose and tap the tendons below the patella.

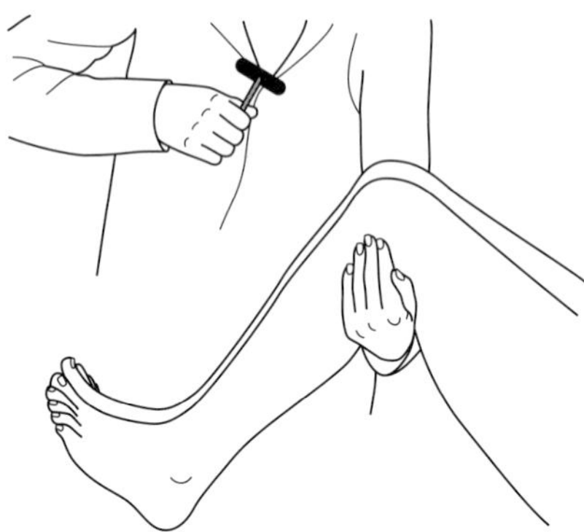

Testing the knee reflexes

- **Ankle reflex (root S1, S2):** by flexing the knee and abducting the leg. Apply gentle pressure to the ball of the foot, with it at a right angle and tap the tendon.

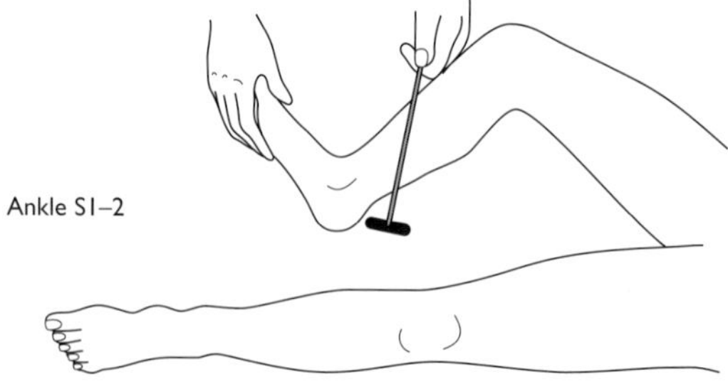

Testing the ankle jerk

Ankle jerks are often absent in the elderly.

- **Compare sides** (right versus left; arms versus legs).

It is essential for the patient to relax and this is not always easy, particularly in the elderly.

Increased jerks—*upper motor neuron lesion* (e.g. hemiparesis).

Decreased jerks—*lower motor neuron lesion* or *acute upper motor neuron lesion*. Need to confirm using 'reinforcement or distraction'. Get the patient to clench

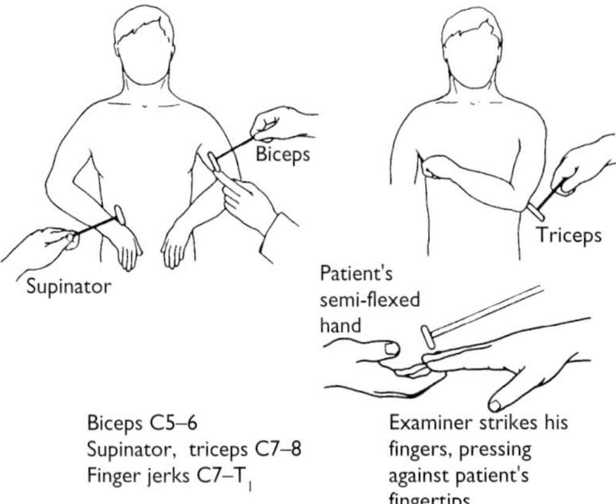

their teeth or pull their hands when you say 'now' and hit the tendon at the same time

Clonus—pressure stretching a muscle group causes rhythmical involuntary contraction. If a brisk reflex is obtained, test for clonus. A sharp, then sustained dorsiflexion of the foot by pressure on the ball of the foot may result in the foot 'beating' for many seconds. Clonus confirms an increased tendon jerk and suggests an *upper motor neuron lesion*. A few symmetrical beats may be normal.

Plantar reflexes

- **Tell patient what you are doing, and scratch the side of the sole with a noxious but not injurious implement.** An orange stick is quite useful. Watch for flexion or extension of the toes.

Normal plantar responses—flexion of all toes.

Extensor (Babinski) response—slow extension of the big toe with spreading of the other toes. Withdrawal from pain or

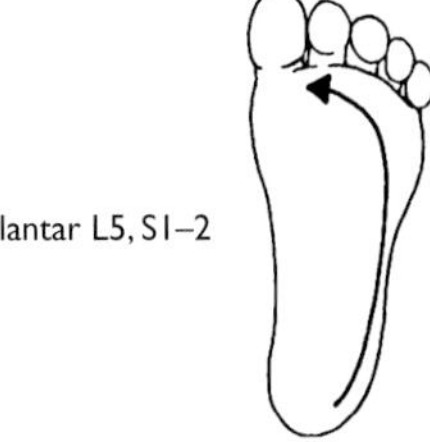

Plantar response stimulus

tickle is rapid and not abnormal. In individuals with sensitive feet, the reflex can be elicited by noxious stimuli elsewhere in the leg; stroking the lateral aspect of the foot can be very useful, or testing pinprick sensation on the dorsum of the great toe.

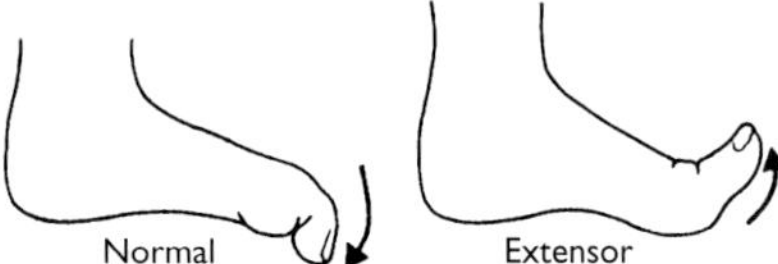

Trunk

- **The superficial abdominal reflexes rarely need to be tested.**
  - Lightly stroke each quadrant with an orange-stick or the back of your fingernail. These reflexes are absent or decreased in an upper or lower motor neuron lesion. They are typically absent in multiple sclerosis.
- **Cremasteric reflex T12–L1.**
  - Not routinely examined. Stroke inside of leg—induces testis to rise from cremaster muscle contraction.
- **Palpate the bladder.**

The patient with a distended bladder will feel very uncomfortable as you palpate it.

Many neurological lesions, sensory or motor, will lead to a distended bladder, giving the patient *retention with overflow incontinence*.

- Examine the strength of the abdominal muscles by asking the patient to attempt to sit up without using their hands.

Sensation

If there are no grounds to expect sensory loss, sensation can be rapidly examined.

Briefly examine each extremity. Success depends on making the patient understand what you are doing.

Children are the best sensory witnesses and dons the worst. The examination is very subjective. As in the motor examination, one is looking for patterns of loss, e.g. nerve root (dermatome), nerve, sensory level (spinal cord), glove/ stocking (peripheral neuropathy), dissociation (i.e. pain and temperature versus vibration and proprioception—e.g. syringomyelia).

Vibration sense

- **Test vibration sense** using a 128/s tuning fork. Place the fork on the sternum first so that the patient appreciates what vibration is. Then place the tuning fork distally on each extremity. The patient should feel the sensation for as long as the examiner (assuming the examiner is normal!). The occasional patient will claim to feel vibration when it is absent—if this is suspected, try a non-vibrating tuning fork; if they feel it vibrate, testing is not valid. Vibration often diminishes with age, probably as part of age-related neuropathy.

Position sense—proprioception

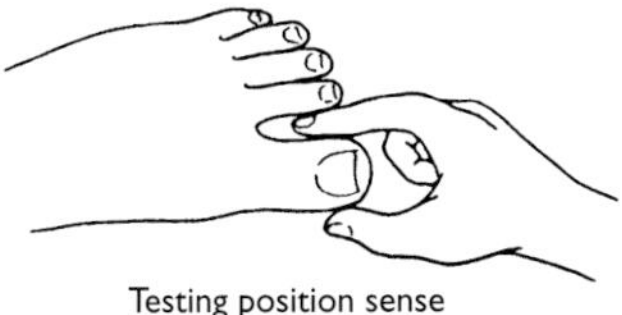

Testing position sense

- Show the patient what you are doing. 'I am going to move your finger/toe up or down' [doing so]. I want you to tell me up or down each time I move it. Now close your eyes.'
- Hold distal to joint, and side to side, with your forefinger and thumb, and make small movements in an irregular, not alternate, sequence, e.g. up, up, down, down, up, down.

Normal threshold is very low—the smallest, slowest passive movement you can produce in the terminal phalanges should always be correctly detected.

Pain

- Take a sterile pin and do not re-use the same pin on another patient.
- Touch the sharp end on the skin. Do not draw blood. Patient's eyes can be open. Usually start on an area you know will be intact, e.g. sternum.
- 'Does this feel sharp, like a pinprick?'

If you find sensory loss, map out that area by proceeding from abnormal to normal area of skin.

If you are uncertain about sensory loss, another (cumbersome) method is to ask the patient to close their eyes, and put either the blunt or sharp end of the pin on the skin in an irregular pattern and ask which is which.

Light touch

- Close patient's eyes.
- 'Say "yes" when I touch you with tactile filaments, 1 g, 10 g and 75 g pressure, or a wisp of cotton wool.' Touch at irregular intervals. Compare sides of body.

Thermal sensation is not examined routinely. Tests with hot and cold water in glass tubes cannot be standardised. Find an area where hot is called cold or vice versa and draw the tube along the skin until true temperature is recognised.

Two-point discrimination. Normal threshold on the fingertip is 2 mm. If sensory impairment is peripheral or in the cord, a raised threshold is found, e.g. 5 mm. If cortical, no threshold is found.

Stereognosis is tested by placing coins, keys, pen top, etc. in the patient's hand and, with eyes closed, the patient attempts to identify by feeling.

Sensory inattention is best found with a pin, not touch. Bilateral simultaneous symmetrical pinpricks are felt only on the normal side, while each is felt if applied separately. Found in cortical lesions.

Dermatomes

Most are easily detected with a pin. Map out from the area of impaired sensation.

Note in arms: **middle finger—C7** and dermatomes either side symmetrical up to mid upper arm.

Note in legs: **lateral border of foot and heel (S1)**, back of legs and anal region have sacral supply.

Some other important dermatomes are C6 median nerve 1st digit (thumb), C7 (radial nerve) 2nd and 3rd fingers, C8 (ulnar nerve) 4th and 5th fingers, T4 nipples, T6 xiphoid, T10 Umbilicus, T12 pubic area.

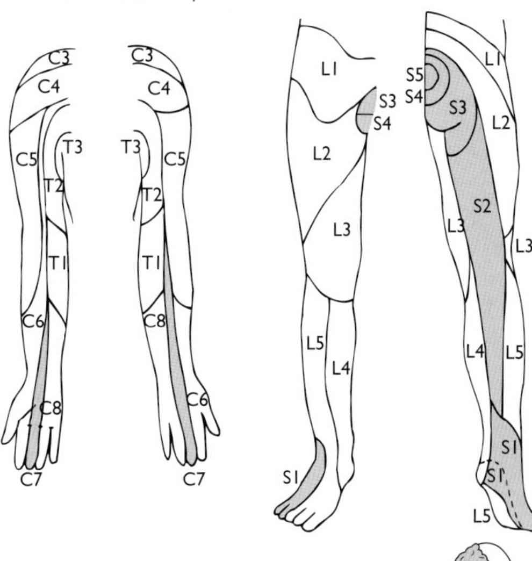

Gait (see Chapter 2)

- **Observe the patient as they walk in. If ataxia is suspected but not seen on ordinary walking, ask the patient to do heel-to-toe walking. (Demonstrate it yourself.)**

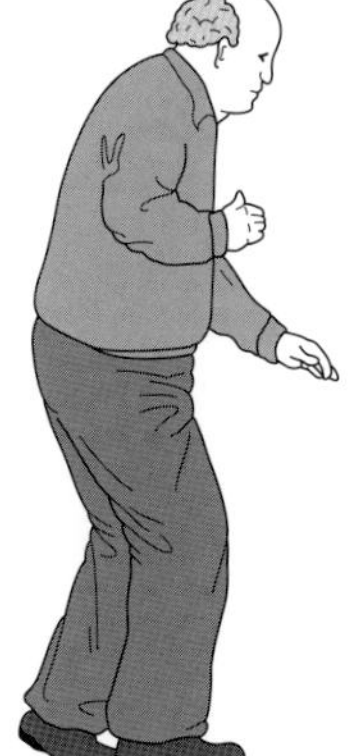

There are many examples of abnormal gait.

Parkinson's disease. Stooped posture with most joints flexed, with small shuffling steps without swinging arms; tremor of hands.

Spastic gait. Scraping toe on one or both sides as patient walks, moving foot in lateral arc to prevent this.

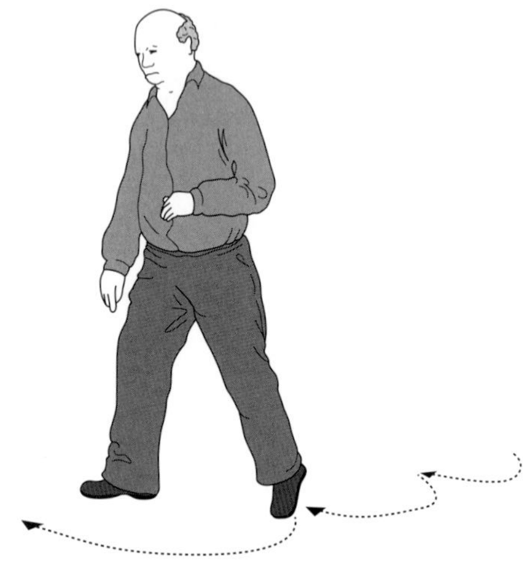

Sensory ataxia. High stepping gait, with slapping-down of feet. Seen with peripheral neuropathy.

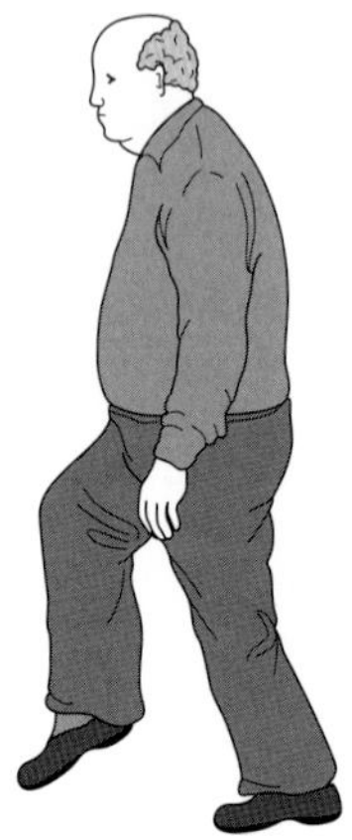

Cerebellar gait. Feet wide apart as patient walks.

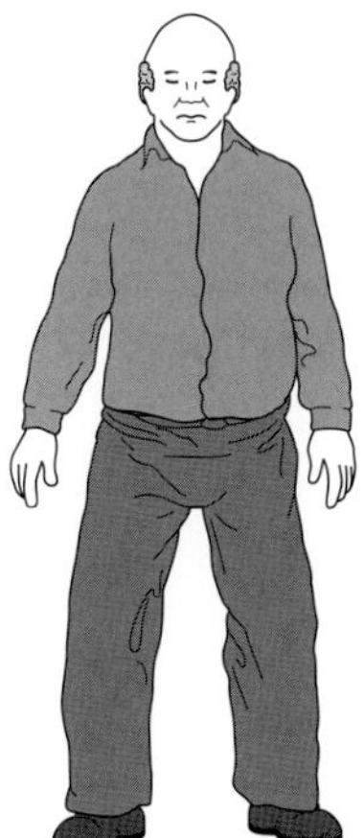

Foot drop. Toe scrapes on ground in spite of excessive lifting-up of leg on affected side.

Shuffling gait. Multiple little steps—typical of diffuse cerebral vascular disease.

Hysterical gait. Usually wild lurching without falling.

Romberg's test is often performed at this time but is mainly a test of position sense. Ask the patient to stand upright with their feet together and close their eyes. If there is any falling noted, the test is positive.

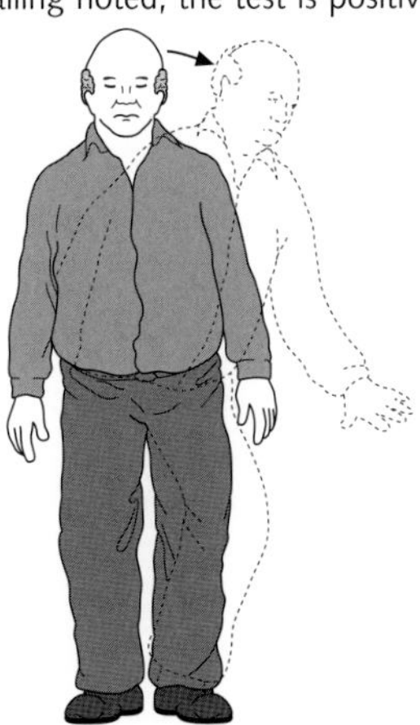

Elderly patients may fail this test and *hysterics* may fall sideways but stop just before they topple over. Test positive with posterior column loss of *tabes dorsalis of syphilis*. Anxious patients may sway excessively; try distracting by testing stereognosis at the same time—the excess swaying may disappear!

Background information

Dorsal column loss of sensation

- Decreased position, vibration and deep pain sensation (squeeze Achilles' tendon).
- Touch often not lost, as half carried in anterior column.

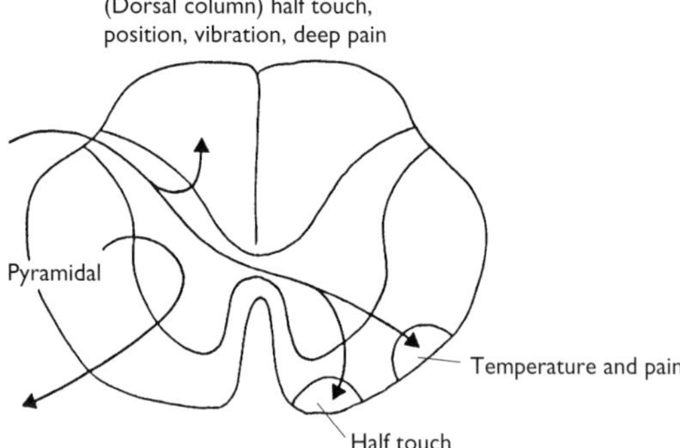

Cortical loss of sensation

Defect shown by deficient:

- position sense
- tactile discrimination
- sensory inattention.

Signs of meningeal irritation

- Neck rigidity—try to flex neck. Resistance or pain? Remember to check for tonsillitis.
- Kernig's sign—not as sensitive as neck rigidity.

Straight-leg-raising for sciatica

- Lift straight leg until pain in back. Then slightly lower until no pain and then dorsiflex foot to 'stretch' sciatic nerve until there is pain.

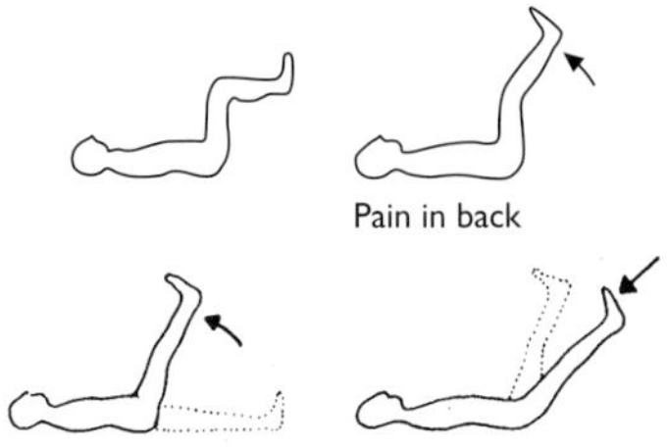

Summary of common illnesses

Lower motor neuron lesion

- wasting
- fasciculation
- hypotonia
- power diminished
- absent reflexes
- ± sensory loss

T1 palsy—weakness of intrinsic muscles of hand: finger abduction and adduction, thumb abduction (cf. median nerve palsy and ulnar nerve palsy)

- sensory loss: medial forearm

median nerve palsy—abductor pollicis brevis weakness (other thenar muscles may be weak)—test opposition of thumb and little finger

- sensory loss: thumb, first two fingers, palmar surface

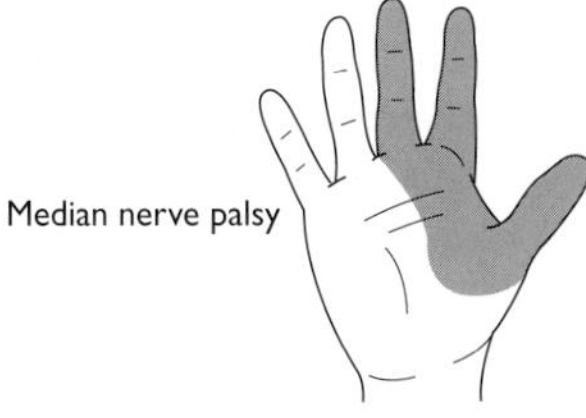

ulnar nerve palsy—interversion, hypothenar muscles wasted, weakness of finger abduction and adduction; claw-hand, cannot extend fingers

- sensory loss: half fourth, all fifth fingers, palmar surface (Figure 7.3)

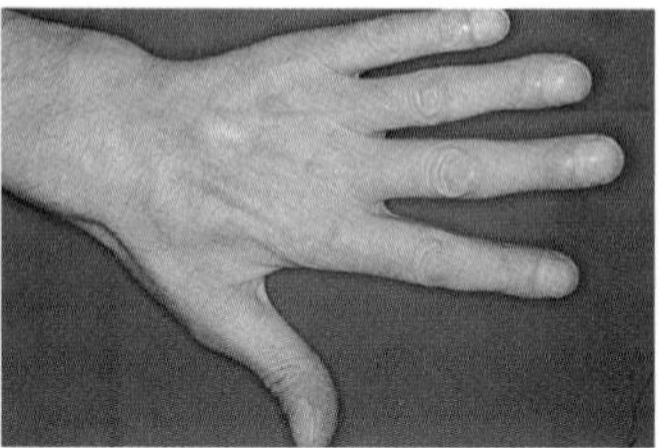

Figure 7.3 Wasted interossei and hypothenar eminence from an ulna nerve or T_1 lesion.

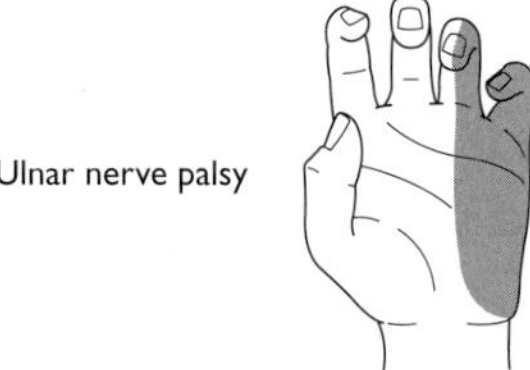

radial nerve palsy—wrist drop

- sensory loss: small area/dorsal web of thumb

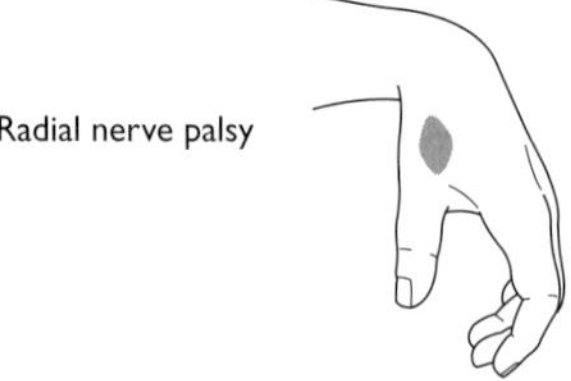

L5 palsy—foot drop and weak inversion; sensory loss on medial aspect of foot
peroneal nerve palsy—foot drop and weak eversion; minor sensory loss of dorsum of foot
S1 palsy—cannot stand on toes, sensory loss of lateral aspect of foot, absent ankle reflex

Upper motor neuron lesion

- no wasting
- extended arms with palms up—hand drifts down
- overswing when hands are tapped

- rapid alternating movements performed slowly: clumsy 'piano playing'
- hypertonia
  - spastic flexion of upper limbs, extension of lower limbs
  - clasp knife
- power diminished
- increased tendon reflexes (± clonus)
- extensor plantar response—classically use orange stick or keys (never the end of the tendon hammer!) —may be elicited by pressure on lateral border of foot, pressure on shin or even on tapping patella
- ± sphincter disturbance
- spastic gait
  - extended stiff leg with foot drop
  - arm does not swing, held flexed

N.B. Check 'level' first, then pathology.

Cerebellar dysfunction

- no wasting
- hypotonia with overswing; irregularity of movements
- intention tremor
- inability to execute rapid alternating movements smoothly (dysdiadochokinesia)
- ataxic gait
- nystagmus
- scanning or staccato speech
- incoordination not improved by sight (whereas is with sensory defect)

Extrapyramidal dysfunction—Parkinson's disease

Bradykinesia, rigidity, tremor and postural instability are the cardinal features:

- flexed posture of body, neck, arms and legs
- expressionless, impassive facies, staring eyes
- 'pill-rolling' tremor of hands at rest
- delay in initiating movements

- tone—'lead pipe' rigidity, possibly with 'cog-wheeling'
- normal power and sensation
- speech quiet and monotonal
- gait—shuffling small steps, possibly with difficulty starting or stopping
- postural instability: test by having patient standing comfortably. Stand behind the patient and give a sharp tug backwards. Normal patients should show a slight sway; taking steps backwards, particularly multiple steps, is abnormal

Multiple sclerosis

- **evidence of 'different lesions in space and time' from history and examination. Usually affects cerebral white matter.** Common sites:
  - optic atrophy—optic neuritis
  - nystagmus—vestibular or cerebellar tracts
  - brisk jaw jerk—pyramidal lesion above fifth nerve
- cerebellar signs in arms or gait—cerebellar tracts
- upper motor neuron signs in arms or legs—pyramidal, right or left (absent superficial abdominal reflexes)
- transverse myelitis with sensory level—indicates level of lesion
- urine retention—usually sensory tract
- sensory perception loss—sensory tract

System-oriented examination

'Examine the higher cerebral functions'

- general appearance
- consciousness level
- mood
- speech
- cognitive
  - confusion
  - orientation
  - attention/calculation
  - memory—short-term, long-term
  - reasoning—understanding of proverb

'Examine the cranial nerves'

I	smell (only test if the hint of smell bottles are present)
II	visual acuity visual fields fundi
III, IV, VI	ptosis nystagmus eye movements pupils
V	sensory face corneal reflex jaw muscles/jerk
VII	face muscles—upper/lower motor neuron defect (taste if taste bottles are provided)
VIII	hearing Rinne/Weber tests nystagmus
IX, X	palate swallowing (taste—posterior third of tongue)
XI	trapezius
XII	tongue wasting

'Examine the arms neurologically'

- *inspect*:
  - abnormal position
  - wasting
  - fasciculation
  - tremor/athetosis
- ask patient to extend arms in front, palms up, keep them there with eyes closed, then check:
  - posture/drift
  - tap back of wrists to assess whether position is stable
  - fast finger movements (pyramidal)
  - touch nose (coordination)—finger–nose test
  - 'Hold my fingers. Pull me up. Push me away'
- tone

- muscle power—each group if indicated
- reflexes
- sensation
  - light touch
  - pinprick
  - vibration
  - proprioception

'Examine the legs neurologically'

- *inspect*:
  - abnormal positions
  - wasting
  - fasciculation
- 'Lift one leg off the bed'
- 'Lift other leg off the bed'
- coordination—heel–toe
- tone
- power—'Pull up toes. Push down toes'
- reflexes
- plantar reflexes
- sensation (as hands)
- Romberg test
- gait and tandem gait

'Examine the arms or legs'

- *inspect*:
  - colour
  - skin/nail changes (Figure 7.4)

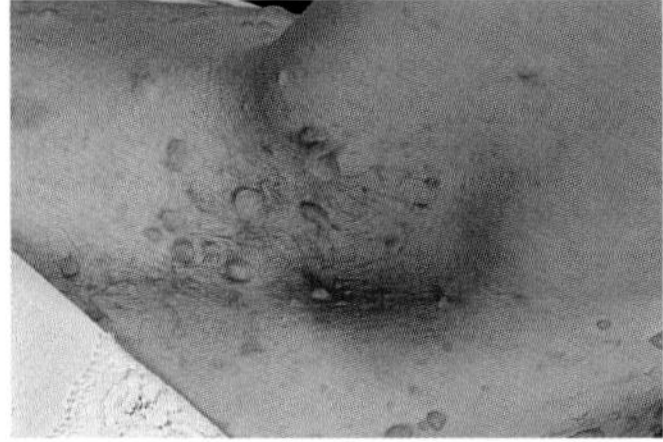

Figure 7.4 Neurofibromatosis Type 1 (von Recklinghausen's disease)—multiple cutaneous fibroma.

    - ulcers
    - wasting (are both arms and legs involved?)
    - joints
- palpate:
    - temperature, pulses
    - lumps (see above)
    - joints
        - active movements
        - feel for crepitus, e.g. hand over knee during flexion
        - passive movements (do not hurt patient)
    - reflexes
    - sensation

CHAPTER 8

Assessment of disability including care of the elderly

Introduction

It is important, particularly in the elderly, to **assess whether the patient has a disability**:

- which interferes with normal life and aspirations
- which makes the patient dependent on others:
  - requires temporary assistance for specific problems
  - occasional or regular assistance long term
  - supervised accommodation
  - nursing home with 24-hour care.

It is necessary to assess the following in a patient:

- **ability to do day-to-day functions**
- **mental ability, including confusion or dementia**
- **emotional state and drive**.

The descriptive terms used for disability have specific definitions in a World Health Organization classification.

- **Impairment**—any loss or abnormality of anatomical, physiological or psychological function, i.e. **systems or parts of the body that do not work**.
- **Disability**—any restrictions or lack of ability (due to an impairment) to perform an activity within the range considered normal, i.e. **activities that cannot be done**.
- **Handicap**—a limitation of normal occupation because of impairment or disability, i.e. **social consequences**.

Clinical Skills and Examination: The Core Curriculum. By R Turner, B Angus, A Handa, C Hatton. ©2009 Blackwell Publishing, ISBN: 9781405157513.

Thus:

- **a hemiparesis is an impairment**
- **an inability to wash or dress is a disability**
- **an inability to do an occupation is a handicap.**

The introductory clinical training in the first few chapters of this book concentrates on evaluation of impairments. Disability and handicap are not always given due attention and are the practical and social aspects of the disease process. It is a mistake if the doctor is preoccupied by impairments, since the patient often perceives disability as the major problem.

The impairments, disability and handicap should have been covered in a normal history and examination, but it can be helpful to bring together important facts to provide an overall assessment.

A summary description of a patient may include the following.

- **Aetiology**—familial hypercholesterolaemia.
- **Pathology**
  - atheroma
  - right middle cerebral artery thrombosis.
- **Impairment**
  - left hemiparesis
  - paralysed left arm, fixed in flexion
  - upper motor neuron signs in left arm and face.
- **Disability**—difficulty during feeding. Cannot drive car.
- **Handicap**
  - can no longer work as a travelling salesman
  - embarrassed to socialise.
- **Social circumstances**—partner can cope with day-to-day living, but lack of income from occupation and withdrawal from society present major problems.

Assessment of impairment

The routine history and examination will often reveal impairments. Additional standard clinical measures are often used to assist quantitation, for example:

- treadmill exercise test
- peak flowmeter
- Medical Research Council scale of muscle power
- making five-pointed star from matches (to detect dyspraxia in hepatic encephalopathy).

Questionnaires can similarly provide a semi-quantitative index of important aspects of impairment and give a brief shorthand description of a patient. The role of the questionnaire is in part a checklist to make sure the key questions are asked.

Cognitive function

In the elderly, impaired cognitive function can be assessed by a standard 10-point **mental test score** introduced by Hodkinson. The test assumes normal communication skills. One mark each is given for correct answers to 10 standard questions:

- age of patient
- time (to nearest hour)
- address given, for recall at end of test, e.g. 42 West Street or 92 Columbia Road
- recognise two people
- year (if January, the previous year is accepted)
- name of place, e.g. hospital or area of town if at home
- date of birth of patient
- start of First World War
- name of monarch in UK, president in US
- count backwards from 20 to 1 (no errors allowed unless self-corrected)
- (check recall of address).

This scale is a basic test of gross defects of memory and orientation and is designed to detect cognitive impairment. It has the advantages of brevity, relative lack of culture-specific knowledge and widespread use. In the elderly, 8–10 is normal, 7 is probably normal, 6 or below is abnormal.

Specific problems, such as confusion or wandering at night, are not included in the mental test score and indicate that the score is a useful checklist but not a substitute for a clinical assessment.

Affect and drive

Motivation is an important determinant of successful rehabilitation. Depression, accompanied by lack of motivation, is a major cause of disability.

Enquire about symptoms of depression and relevant examination (see Chapter 1, Mental state), e.g. 'How is your mood? Have you lost interest in things?'

Making appropriate lifestyle changes, recruiting help from friends or relatives, can be key to increasing motivation. Pharmaceutical treatment of depression can also be helpful.

Assessment of disability

Assessing restrictions to daily activities is often the key to successful management.

- **Make a list of disabilities separate from other problems, e.g. diagnoses, symptoms, impairments, social problems.**

This list can assist with setting priorities, including which investigations or therapies are most likely to be of benefit to the patient.

Activities of daily living (ADL)

These are key functions which in the elderly affect the degree of independence. Several scales of disability have been used. One of these, the **Barthel index of ADL**, records the following disabilities that can affect self-care and mobility:

- continence—urinary and faecal
- ability to use toilet
- grooming
- feeding
- dressing
- bathing
- transfer, e.g. chair to bed
- walking
- using stairs.

The assessment denotes the current state and not the underlying cause or the potential improvement. It does not include cognitive functions or emotional state. It emphasises independence, so a catheterised patient who can competently manage the device achieves the full score for urinary incontinence. The total score provides an overall estimate or summary of dependence, but between-patient comparisons are difficult as they may have different combinations of disability. Interpretation of score depends on disability and facilities available.

Instrumental activities of daily living (IADL)

These are slightly more complex activities relating to an individual's ability to live independently. They often require special assessment in the home environment:

- preparing a meal
- doing light housework
- using transport
- managing money
- shopping
- doing laundry
- taking medications
- using a telephone.

Communication

In the elderly, difficulty in communication is a frequent problem, and impairment of the following may need special attention:

- deafness (do the ears need syringing? Is a hearing aid required?)
- speech (is dysarthria due to lack of teeth?)
- an alarm to call for help when required
- aids for reading, e.g. spectacles, magnifying glass
- resiting or adaptation of doorbell, telephone, radio or television.

Analysing disabilities and handicaps and setting objectives

After writing a list of disabilities, it is necessary to make a possible treatment plan with specific

objectives. The plan needs to be realistic. A multidisciplinary team approach, including social workers, physiotherapists, occupational therapists, nurses and doctors is usually essential in rehabilitation of elderly patients.

The overall aims in treating the elderly include the following.

- To make diagnoses, if feasible, particularly to treatable illnesses.
- To comfort and alleviate problems and stresses, even if one cannot cure.
- To add life to years, even if one cannot add years to life.

Specific aspects that may need attention include the following.

- Alleviate social problems if feasible.
- Improve heating, clothing, toilet facilities, cooking facilities.
- Arrange support services, e.g. help with shopping, provision of meals, attendance at day centre.
- Arrange regular visits from nurse or other helper.
- Make sure family, neighbours and friends understand the situation.
- Treat depression.
- Help with sorting out finances.
- Provide aids, for example:
  - large-handled implements
  - walking frame or stick
  - slip-on shoes
  - handles by bath or toilet.
- Help to keep as mobile as feasible.
- Facilitate visits to hearing-aid centre, optician, chiropodist, dentist.
- Ensure medications are kept to a minimum, and the instructions and packaging are suitable.

A major problem is if the disability leads to the patient being unwelcome. This depends on the reactions of others and requires tactful discussion with all concerned.

Identifying causes for disabilities

Specific disabilities may have specific causes which can be alleviated. In the elderly, common problems include the following.

Confusion

This is an impairment. Common causes are:

- infection
- drugs
- other illnesses, e.g. heart failure
- sensory deprivation, e.g. deafness, darkness.

Assume all confusion is an acute response to an unidentified cause.

Incontinence

- toilet far away, e.g. upstairs
- physical restriction of gait
- urine infection
- faecal impaction
- uterine prolapse
- diabetes

'Off legs'

- neurological impairment
- unsuspected fracture of leg
- depressed
- general illness, e.g. infection, heart failure, renal failure, hypothermia, hypothyroid, diabetes, hypokalaemia

Falls

- insecure carpet
- dark stairs
- poor vision, e.g. cataracts
- postural hypotension
- cardiac arrhythmias
- epilepsy
- neurological deficit, e.g. Parkinson's disease, hemiparesis
- cough or micturition syncope
- intoxication

CHAPTER 9
Basic examination, notes and diagnostic principles

Basic examination

In practice, one cannot attempt to elicit every single physical sign for each system. Basic signs should be sought on every examination, and if there is any hint of abnormality, additional physical signs can be elicited to confirm the suspicion. Listed below are the basic examinations of the systems which will enable you to complete a routine examination adequately but not excessively.

- **General examination**
  - general appearance
  - is the patient well, ill or very ill?
  - look at temperature chart or take patient's temperature
  - any obvious abnormality?
  - mental state, mood, behaviour
- **General and cardiovascular system**
  - observation—dyspnoea, distress
  - blood pressure
  - hands
    - temperature
    - nails, e.g. clubbing, liver palms
  - pulse—rate, rhythm, character
  - axillae—lymph nodes
  - neck—lymph nodes, masses
  - face and eyes—anaemia, jaundice, xanthelasma

Clinical Skills and Examination: The Core Curriculum. By R Turner, B Angus, A Handa, C Hatton. ©2009 Blackwell Publishing, ISBN: 9781405157513.

- tongue and fauces—central cyanosis
- jugular venous pressure (JVP)—height and waveform
- apex beat—position and character
- parasternal—heave or thrills
- stethoscope
  - heart sounds, added sounds, murmurs
  - listen in all four areas with stethoscope diaphragm
  - lie patient on left side, bell of stethoscope—mitral stenosis (MS)
  - sit patient up, lean forward, breathe out—aortic incompetence (AI)

- **Respiratory system**
  - observation
  - trachea—position
  - **front of chest**
    - movement
    - percuss—compare sides
    - auscultate
  - **back of chest**
    - movement
    - percuss—particularly level of bases
    - auscultate
  - examine sputum
- **Examine spine**
- **Abdomen**
  - lie patient flat
  - feel femoral pulses and inguinal lymph nodes
  - herniae
  - look at abdomen—ask if pain or tenderness
  - palpate abdomen gently
    - generally all over? Masses
    - abdominal aorta
    - liver—then percuss
    - spleen—then percuss
    - kidneys
    - (ascites if indicated)
  - (auscultate if indicated)
  - males—genitals

- per rectum (PR; only if given permission)—usually at end of examination
- per vaginam (PV)—rarely by student

- **Legs**
  - observation
  - arterial pulses (joints if indicated)
  - neurology:

• reflexes	• knees • ankles • plantar responses	tone power coordination	only if indicated
• sensation	• pinprick • vibration	position cotton wool temperature	only if indicated

- **Arms**
  - posture: outstretched hands, eyes closed, rapid finger movements
  - finger–nose coordination:

• reflexes	• triceps • biceps • supinator	tone power	only if indicated
• sensation	• pinprick	vibration position cotton-wool temperature	only if indicated

- **Cranial nerves**
  - I (if indicated)
  - II: eyes —reading print
    - pupils—torch and accommodation
    - ophthalmoscope—fundi
    - fields
  - III, IV, VI: eye movements—'Do you see double?'

note nystagmus

- V, VII – open mouth
  - grit teeth—feel masseters
  - sensation—cotton wool
  - (corneal reflex—if indicated)
  - (taste—if indicated)

  - VIII: hearing—watch at each ear
    - (Rinne, Weber tests if indicated)
  - IX, X: fauces movement
  - XI: shrug shoulders
  - XII: put out tongue
- **Walk**—look at gait
- **Herniae and varicose veins**

Example of notes

Record keeping is essential and needs to be accurate and contemporaneous.

Every sheet in the patient's notes MUST have the patient's name and date of birth and/or hospital number in the top right-hand corner.

Patient's name: Age: Occupation:
Date of admission/Clerking and time
Complains of:

- list, in patient's words

History of present illness:

- detailed description of each symptom (even if appears irrelevant)
- last well
- chronological order, with both actual date of onset and time previous to admission
- (may include history from informant—in which case, state this is so)
- then detail other questions that seem relevant to possible differential diagnoses
- then **functional enquiry**, 'check' system for other symptoms
- (minimal statement in notes—weight, appetite, digestion, bowels, micturition, menstruation, if appropriate)

Past history:

- chronological order

Family history:

Personal and social history:

- must include details of home circumstances, dependants, patient's occupation
- effect of illness on life and its relevance to foreseeable discharge of patient smoking, alcohol, drug misuse

Drug history:

- including drug allergies

Physical examination:

- general appearance, etc.
- then record findings according to systems

Minimal statement:

Healthy, well-nourished woman.
Afebrile, not anaemic, icteric or cyanosed.
No enlargement of lymph nodes.
No clubbing.
Breasts and thyroid normal.

Cardiovascular system (CVS):	Blood pressure, pulse rate and rhythm. JVP not raised. Apex position. Heart sounds 1 and 2, no murmurs.
Respiratory system:	Chest and movements normal. Percussion note normal. Breath sounds vesicular. No other sounds.
Abdominal system:	Tongue and fauces normal. Abdomen normal, no tenderness. Liver, spleen, kidneys, bladder impalpable. No masses felt. Hernial orifices normal. Rectal examination normal or not done

Vaginal examination not performed.
Testes normal.

Central nervous system (CNS):	Alert and intelligent.		
	Pupils equal, regular, react equally to light and accommodation.		
	Fundi normal.		
	Normal eye movements.		
	Other cranial nerves normal.		
	Limbs normal.		
	Biceps jerks	+	+
	Triceps jerks	+	+
	Supinator jerk	+	+
	Knee jerks	+	+
	Ankle jerks	+	+
	Plantar reflexes	↓	↓
	Touch and vibration normal.		
	Spine and joints normal.		
	Gait normal.		

Pulses (including dorsalis pedis and posterior tibial) palpable.

Summary

Write a few sentences only:

- salient positive features of history and examination
- relevant negative information
- home circumstances
- patient's medical state
  - understanding of illness
  - specific concerns

State your name and designation, e.g. A Bloggs, SHO medicine, and a contact number, e.g. Bleep

Problem list and diagnoses

After your history and examination, **make a list of**:

- **the diagnoses you have been able to make**
- **problems or abnormal findings that need explaining**.

For example:

- symptoms or signs

- anxiety
- poor social background
- laboratory results
- drug sensitivities.

It is best to separate the current problems of actual or potential clinical significance requiring treatment or follow-up, from the inactive problems. An example is:

Active problems	**Date**
1 Unexplained episodes of fainting	1 week
2 Angina	since 1990
3 Hypertension—blood pressure 190/100 mmHg	1990
4 Chronic renal failure—plasma creatinine 200 μmol/l	August 1996
5 Widower, unemployed, lives on own	
6 Anxious about possibility of being injured in a fall	
7 Smokes 40 cigarettes per day	

Inactive problems	**Date**
1 Thyrotoxicosis treated by partial thyroidectomy	1976
2 ACE inhibitor-induced cough	1991

At first you will have difficulty knowing which problems to put down separately, and which can be covered under one diagnosis and a single entry. It is therefore advisable to rewrite the problem list if a problem resolves or can be explained by a diagnosis. When you have some experience, it will be appropriate to fill out the problems on a complete problem list at the front of the notes:

Active problems	Date	Inactive problems	Date
Include symptoms, signs, unexplained abnormal investigations, social and psychiatric problems		Include major past illness, operation or hypersensitivities. Do not include problems requiring active care	

From the problem list, you should be able to make:

- **differential diagnoses**, including that which you think is most likely. Remember:
  - **common diseases occur commonly**
  - **an unusual manifestation of a common disease** is more likely than an uncommon disease
  - when you hear hoof beats, think of horses, not zebras
  - **do not necessarily be put off by some aspect which does not fit** (What is the farmer's friend that has four legs, wags its tail and says 'cockadoodledoo'? A dog, and the sound was from another animal)
- **possible diagnostic investigations** you feel are appropriate
- **management and therapy** you think are appropriate
- **prognostic implications.**

Diagnoses

The diagnostic terms that physicians use often relate to different levels of understanding.

Disordered function	Immobile painful joint	Breathlessness	Angina
	↑	↑	↑
Structural lesion	Osteoarthritis	Anaemia	Narrow coronary artery
	↑	↑	↑
Pathology	Iron-deposition fibrosis (haemochromatosis)	Iron deficiency	Aortitis
	↑	↑	↑
Aetiology	Inherited disorder of iron metabolism—homozygous for C282Y with A-H	Bleeding duodenal ulcer	*Treponema pallidum* (syphilis)

Different problems require diagnoses at different levels, which may change as further information becomes available. Thus, a patient on admission may be diagnosed as *pyrexia of unknown origin*. After a plain X-ray of the abdomen, he may be found to have a *renal mass*, which on a computed tomographic (CT) scan becomes *perinephric abscess*, which from blood cultures is found to be *Staphylococcus aureus* infection. For a complete diagnosis all aspects should be known, but often this is not possible.

Note many terms are used as a diagnosis but, in fact, cover considerable ignorance, e.g. *diabetes mellitus* (originally 'sweet-tasting urine', but now also diagnosed by high plasma glucose) is no more than a descriptive term of disordered function. *Sarcoid* relates to a pattern of symptoms and a pathology of non-caseating granulomata, of which the aetiology is unknown.

Progress notes

While the patient is in hospital, full progress notes should be kept to give a complete picture of:

- how the diagnosis was established
- how the patient was treated
- the evolution of the illness
- any complications that occurred.

These notes are as important as the account of the original examination. In acute cases, record daily changes in signs and symptoms. In chronic cases, the relevant systems should be re-examined at least once a week and the findings recorded.

It is useful to separate different aspects of the illness:

- symptoms
- signs
- laboratory investigations
- general assessment, e.g. apparent response to therapy
- further plans, which would include educating the patient and their family about the illness.

Objective findings such as alterations in weight, improvement in colour, temperature, pulse, character of respirations or fluid intake and output are more valuable than purely **subjective statements** such as 'feeling better' or 'slept well'.

When appropriate, daily observations, e.g. blood pressure readings or analyses of the urine, should be recorded.

An account of all ward procedures such as aspirations of chest should be included.

Specifically record:

- the findings and comments of the physician or surgeon in charge
- results of a case conference
  - an opinion from another department
  - ALL encounters with the patient should be recorded. If it is not in the notes, it did not happen in the eyes of the law. Thus all ward rounds should be recorded.

Problem-oriented records

Dr Larry Weed proposed a system of note keeping in which the history and examination constituted a database. All subsequent notes are structured according to the **specific numbered problems** in a problem list. Problem-oriented records really require a special system of note keeping. The full system is therefore not often used, but the problem list is an extremely valuable check that all aspects of the patient's illness are being covered.

Serial investigations

The results of these should be collected together in a **table** on a special sheet. When any large series of investigations is made, e.g. serial blood counts, erythrocyte sedimentation rates or multiple biochemical analyses, the results can also be expressed by a **graph**.

Operation notes

In patients undergoing surgical treatment, an operation note must be written immediately after the operation. Do not trust your memory for any length of time as several similar problems may be operated on at one session. Even if you are distracted by an emergency, the notes must be written up the same day as the operation. These notes should contain definite statements on the following facts:

- patient name, date of birth and hospital number
- name of surgeon performing the operation and his assistant
- date of procedure
- name of anaesthetist and anaesthetic used
- type and dimension of incision used
- pathological condition found, and mention of anatomical variations
- operative procedures carried out
- any untoward events in the procedure (intraoperative difficulty or variation from standard procedure)
- method of repair of wound and suture materials used
- whether drainage used, material used and whether sutured to wound
- type of dressing used
- postoperative instructions, e.g. frequency of observations, continuing antibiotics, anticoagulation or other special medical or nursing needs.

Postoperative notes

Daily after the operation till discharged:

- the general condition of the patient
- any complication or troublesome symptom, e.g. pain, haemorrhage, vomiting, distension, etc.
- any treatment.

Discharge note

A full statement of the patient's condition on discharge should be written:

- date of admission
- date of discharge
- where discharged to, e.g. home, community hospital, etc.
- diagnosis
- treatment received/procedure undertaken
- active problems
- medication and other therapies
- specific follow-up points, e.g. persistent depressive disorder, blood pressure monitoring
- what the patient has been told
- follow up, i.e. when the patient is next being seen
- an estimate of the prognosis.

If the patient dies, the student must attend a post-mortem and then complete their note by a short account of the autopsy findings.

CHAPTER 10

Presenting cases and communication

Presentations to doctors

Medicine is a subject in which you have to be able to talk, as they say on Radio 4, 'without repetition, hesitation or deviation'. The more practice you get, the better you will become and the more confident you will appear in front of doctors, nurses and patients. Confidence displayed by the doctor is an important aspect of therapy and the value to the patient of a doctor who can speak lucidly is enormous.

Practise talking to yourself in a mirror, avoiding any breaks or interpolating the word 'er'. Open a textbook, find a subject and give a little talk on it to yourself. Even if you do not know anything about the subject, you will be able to make up a few coherent sentences once you are practised.

A presentation is not the time to demonstrate you have been thorough and have asked all questions, but is a time to show you can intelligently assemble the essential facts.

In all presentations, give the salient positive findings and the relevant negative findings.

For example:

- in a patient with progressive dyspnoea, state if patient has ever smoked
- in a patient with icterus, state if patient has not been abroad, has not had any recent injections or drugs, or contact with other jaundiced patients.

Clinical Skills and Examination: The Core Curriculum. By R Turner, B Angus, A Handa, C Hatton. ©2009 Blackwell Publishing, ISBN: 9781405157513.

Three types of presentation are likely to be encountered: presentation of a case to a meeting, presentation of a new case on a ward round and a brief follow-up presentation.

Presentation of a case to a meeting

This must be properly prepared, including visual aids as necessary. The principal details, shown on an overhead projector, are helpful as a reminder to you, and the audience may more easily remember the details of a case if they 'see' as well as 'hear' them.

- Practise your presentation from beginning to end and leave nothing to chance.
- Do not speak to the screen; speak to the audience.
- Do not crack jokes, unless you are confident that they are apposite.
- Do not make sweeping statements.
- Remember what you are advised to do in a court of law—dress up, stand up, speak up, shut up.
- Read up about the disease or problem beforehand so that you can answer any queries.
- Read a recent leading article, review or research publication on the subject.

In many hospitals it is expected that you present a journal review of an **original article**. Be prepared to evaluate and criticise the manuscript. Use evidence-based medicine techniques such as PICO (**P**atients or populations, **I**nterventions, **C**omparison group(s) or 'gold standard', **O**utcome(s) of interest). Assess the **validity**: 'Can I trust this information?'; **clinical importance**: 'If true, will the use of this information make an important difference?'; and **applicability**: 'Can I use the information in this instance?' If your seniors cannot give you references, look up the subject on the internet or in large textbooks, or ask the librarian for advice. Laboriously repeating standard information from a textbook is often a turn-off. A recent series or research paper is more educational for you, and more interesting for the audience. Remember you know most about the patient but not necessarily the topic.

The overhead should summarise any presentation:

Mr AB Age: *x* years Brief description, e.g. occupation

Complains of
(state in patient's words—for *x* period)

History of present complaint
- essential details
- other relevant information, e.g. risk factors
- relevant negative information relating to possible diagnoses
- extent to which symptoms or disease limit normal activity
- other symptoms—mention briefly

Past history
- briefly mention inactive problems
- information about active problems, or inactive problems relevant to present illness
- record allergies, including type of reaction to drugs

Family history
- brief information about parents, otherwise detail only if relevant

Social history
- brief, unless relevant
- give family social background
- occupation and previous occupations
- any other special problems
- tobacco or ethanol abuse, past or present

Treatment
- note all drugs with doses

On examination
General description
- introductory descriptive sentence, e.g. well, obese man

- clinical signs relevant to disease
- relevant negative findings

Remember these findings should be descriptive data rather than your interpretation.

Problem list

Differential diagnoses
(put in order of likelihood)

Investigations
- relevant positive findings
- relevant negative findings
- tables or graphs for repetitive data
- photocopy an electrocardiogram or temperature chart for overhead presentation

Progress report

Plan
Subjects that often are discussed after your presentation are:
- other differential diagnoses
- other features of presumed diagnosis that might have been present or require investigation
- pathophysiological mechanisms
- mechanisms of action of drugs and possible side-effects.

After clinical discussion, be prepared to present a publication with essential details on an overhead.

Presentation of a new case on a ward round

- Good written notes are of great assistance. Do not read your notes word for word—use your notes as a reference.
- Highlight, underline or asterisk key features you wish to refer to, or write up a separate note card for reference.
- Talk formally and avoid speaking too quickly or too slowly. Speak to the whole assembled group rather than a tête-à-tête with the consultant.

- Stand upright—it helps to make you appear confident.
- If you are interrupted by a discussion, note where you are and be ready to resume, repeating the last sentence before proceeding.

History

The format will be similar to that on an overhead, with emphasis on positive findings and relevant negative information. A full description of the initial main symptom is usually required.

Examination

Once your history is complete the consultant may ask for the relevant clinical signs only. Still add in relevant negative signs you think are important.

Summary

Be prepared to give a problem list and differential diagnoses.

If you are presenting the patient at the bedside, ensure the patient is comfortable. If the patient wishes to make an additional point or clarification, it is best to welcome this. If it is relevant it can be helpful. If irrelevant, politely say to the patient you will come back to him in a moment, after you have presented the findings. Do not appear to argue with the patient.

Brief follow-up presentation

Give a brief, orienting introduction to provide a framework on which other information can be placed. For example:

> A *xx*-year-old man who was admitted *xx* days ago.
> Long-standing problems include *xxxxx* (list briefly).
> Presented with *xx* symptoms for *x* period.
> On examination had *xx* signs.
> Initial diagnosis of *xx* was confirmed/supported by/not supported by *xx* investigations.
> He was treated by *xx*.
> Since then *xx* progress:
> - symptoms
> - examination.

Start with general description and temperature chart and, if relevant, investigations.

If there are multiple active problems, describe each separately, for example:

- first in regard to the *xxxx*
- second in regard to the *xxxx*

The outstanding problems are *xxxx*.
The plan is *xxxx*.

Aides-mémoire
These are basic lists that provide brief reminders when presenting patients and diseases. Organising one's thoughts along structured lines is helpful.

History

- principal symptom(s)
- history of present illness: 'How did your illness begin?'
- note chronology
- present situation
- functional enquiry
- past history
- family history
- personal and social history

Pain or other symptoms

- site
- radiation
- character
- severity
- onset/duration
- frequency/periodicity or constant
- precipitating factors
- relieving factors
- associated symptoms
- getting worse or better?

Lumps

- Inspection
  - site

        - size
        - shape
        - surface
        - surroundings
    - Palpation
        - soft/solid consistency
        - surroundings—fixed/mobile
        - tender
        - pulsatility
        - transmission of illumination
    - Local lymph nodes

'Tell me about the disease'

- incidence
- geographical area
- gender/age
- aetiology
- pathology
    - macroscopic
    - microscopic
- pathophysiology
- symptoms
- signs
- therapy
- prognosis

Causes of disease

- **genetic**
- **infective**
    - virus
    - bacterial
    - fungal
    - parasitic
- **neoplastic**
    - cancer
        - primary
        - secondary
    - lymphoma

- **vascular**
  - atheroma
  - hypertension
  - other, e.g. arteritis
- **infiltrative**
  - fibrosis
  - amyloid
  - granuloma
- **autoimmune**
- **endocrine**
- **degenerative**
- **environmental**
  - trauma
  - iatrogenic—drug side-effects
  - poisoning
- **malnutrition**
  - general
  - specific, e.g. vitamin defiency
  - perinatal with effects on subsequent development

Diagnostic labels

- **aetiology, e.g. tuberculosis, genetic**

  ↓
- **pathology, e.g. sarcoid, amyloid**

  ↓
- **disordered function, e.g. hypertension, diabetes**

  ↓
- **symptoms or signs, e.g. jaundice, erythema nodosum**

People—including patients

A significant number of disasters, a great deal of irritation and a lot of unpleasantness could be avoided in hospitals by proper communication. The doctor is not the boss but is part of a team, all of whom significantly help the patient. You must be able to communicate properly with the nursing staff, physiotherapists, occupational therapists, administrators, ancillary staff and, above all, patients.

When you first arrive on the wards it is a good idea to go and see the ward sister, physiotherapist, etc., and find out what their job is, what their difficulties are and how they view the patient, other groups and, most importantly, yourself.

Remember these points.

- **Time**—when you talk to anyone, try not to appear in a rush or they will lose concentration and not listen. A little time taken to talk to somebody properly will help enormously. One minute spent sitting down can seem like 5 minutes to the patient; 5 minutes standing up can seem like 1 minute.
- **Silence**—in normal social interaction we tend to avoid silences. In a conversation, as soon as one person stops talking (or even before) the other person jumps in to say their bit. When interviewing patients, it is often useful, if you wish to encourage the patient to talk further, to remain silent a moment longer than would be natural. An encouraging nod of the head, or an echoing of the patient's last word or two may also encourage the patient to talk further.
- **Listen**—active listening to someone is not easy but is essential for good communication. Many people stop talking but not all appear to be listening. Sitting down with the patient is advantageous, both in helping you to concentrate and in transmitting to the patient that you are willing to listen.
- **Smile**—grumpiness or irritation is the best way to stop a patient talking. A smile will often encourage a patient to tell you problems they would not normally do. It helps everybody to relax.
- **Reassurance**—if you appear confident and relaxed this helps others to feel the same. Being calm without excessive body movements can help. Note how a good consultant has a reassuring word for patients and allows others in the team to feel they are (or are capable of) working effectively. As a student you are not in a position to do this, but you can contribute by

playing your role efficiently and calmly.
- **Humility**—no one, in particular the patient, is inferior to you.

Breaking bad news

Bad news is any information that changes a person's view of the future in a negative way. Physicians frequently must break bad news to patients and their loved ones. Students should not routinely be breaking bad news, however it is useful to understand the basics and in fact these can be the basis for any form of professional communication. The mnemonic SPIKES is a useful way to remember: Setting up, Perception, Invitation, Knowledge, Emotions, Strategy and summary.

Setting up: breaking bad news should be done in private in a quiet area; only the patient and a few relatives, as well as relevant members of the healthcare team, should be present. The physician should sit down, make eye contact with the patient, and use touch appropriately. Sufficient time should be allowed to answer questions. Interruptions (e.g. pagers) should be minimised.

Patient perceptions: physicians need to find out what the patient knows about their illness before breaking bad news. Questions that reveal patient perception include: 'What have you been told about your condition?' and 'Do you recall why we did this test?' Assessing patient perceptions allows physicians to correct misinformation and tailor the news to the patient's level of comprehension.

Invitation to break news: physicians need to get the patient's permission to share bad news. For example, the physician may say, 'I'd like to share with you the results of your tests. Is that okay?' Before ordering tests or procedures, physicians need to inform patients about possible outcomes, which prepares patients for potential bad news. Physicians also should ask patients if they want only basic information or a detailed explanation.

Knowledge: patients need enough information to

make informed healthcare decisions; thus, physicians should convey information at the patient's level of comprehension. For example, the word 'spread' should be used in place of 'metastasised'. To help patients adequately process bad news, small pieces of information should be given. Physicians can check for comprehension by asking, 'Am I making sense?' or 'Can I clarify anything?' Undue bluntness and misleading optimism should be avoided. It is usually unhelpful to give specific time periods regarding prognosis.

Emotions: the empathic physician acknowledges a patient's emotional response to bad news by first identifying the emotion and then responding to it. 'I can see that you are upset by this news' is an empathic statement. Deliberate periods of silence allow patients to process bad news and ventilate emotions.

Strategy and summary: after receiving bad news, a patient may experience a sense of isolation and uncertainty. Physicians can minimise the patient's anxiety by summarising the areas discussed, checking for comprehension, and formulating a strategy and follow-up plan with the patient. Written materials (e.g. hand-written notes or prepared materials listing the diagnosis and treatment options) may be helpful. Physicians should assure the patient of their availability to address symptoms, answer questions, and meet other needs. (Adapted from Mueller MD. *Postgraduate Medicine* 2002; **112** (3))

Use of translators and communicating with deaf patients

The General Medical Council (GMC) requires its doctors to 'Respect the rights of patients to be fully involved in decisions about their care, give patients information in a form they can understand, listen to patients and respect their views, respect patients' dignity and privacy, recognise the limits of your professional competence.'

It is difficult to see how the above can be achieved when doctor and patient do not use the same language.

The GMC standards and ethics committee also made the following statement: 'Make arrangements wherever possible to meet particular language and communication needs, for example, through translations, independent interpreters.'

There are many occasions now when translators need to be used. This includes patients who are deaf and use sign language. There are telephone translation services available for many languages via NHS Direct and most local authorities have a translation service. There are a few points to bear in mind, such as how the cultural environment affects the doctor/patient and translator. For example, a female patient unwilling to discuss personal problems through a male translator: some communities are small and confidentiality may be compromised.

It is important to establish the ground rules with the translator at the start of the consultation.

Written communication

Writing in the notes

Write legibly in ink. If you made a mistake, simply cross out the unwanted part of the sentence with a single horizontal line. Then write 'error' next to or above the corrected area and initial it. Never scribble over any part of the note, or use 'white-out' to cover a mistake. Those who read and examine a medical record must be able to see mistakes and know who is responsible for crossing a word or sentences out. For neatness sake you may want to start at the top of a page and avoid too much (any) blank space above your note. You should also provide room for the doctor to amend and initial your note at the end.

Remember that the medical notes are a legal document, but like everything, you should try to get practice at writing in them as a student. It is important to write your name and designation legibly. One clear way of communicating between teams is by using a standardised format. One method is the SOAP. Complete sentences are not necessary.

The four parts of a SOAP note are outlined below:

- **Subjective**—The initial portion of the SOAP note format consists of subjective observations. These are symptoms the patient verbally expresses or as stated by a significant other. These subjective observations include the patient's descriptions of pain or discomfort, the presence of nausea or dizziness, and a multitude of other descriptions of dysfunction, discomfort or illness the patient describes.
- **Objective**—The next part of the format is the objective observation. These objective observations include symptoms that can actually be measured, such as vital signs (temperature, pulse, respiration, skin colour, swelling) and the results of diagnostic tests.
- **Assessment**—Assessment is the diagnosis of the patient's condition. In some cases the diagnosis may be clear. However, it may be a differential diagnosis. This will usually be the doctor's diagnosis reported by you.
- **Plan**—The plan may include laboratory and/or radiological tests ordered for the patient, medications ordered, treatments performed (e.g. minor surgery procedure), patient referrals (sending patient to a specialist), patient discharge plan (e.g. home care, bed rest, short-term/long-term disability, days excused from work, admission to hospital), patient directions and follow-up directions for the patient, and the involvement of other professionals such as physiotherapists, dieticians, speech and language therapists and occupational therapists.

Telephone communication

It is estimated that around a quarter of all communication between doctors and patients takes place by telephone and that this is responsible for many medical errors. It is important to make notes of when the call took place, who called and the details of the discussion. This should be entered into the medical notes wherever possible. It is very important to preserve patient confidentiality and all identifying details except hospital numbers should be removed if letters are being faxed.

SECTION II

Clinical investigation and practical skills

CHAPTER 11
Clinical and radiological investigations

Introduction

This brief introduction to major clinical investigations starts with a general description of the major techniques, and is followed by an outline of the specialised investigations in various medical fields.

Ultrasound examinations

Ultrasound transducers produce and receive high-frequency ultrasound waves. They are moved over the skin surface to produce images of the underlying organ structures from the reflected sound waves. Structures with very few interfaces, such as fluid-filled structures, allow through transmission of the sound waves and therefore appear more **black** on the screen. Structures with a large number of interfaces cause significant reflection and refraction of the sound waves and therefore appear **whiter**. Air causes almost complete attenuation of the sound wave and therefore structures deep to this cannot be visualised.

Ultrasound scanning is a real-time examination and is dependent on the experience of the operator for its accuracy. The diagnosis is made from the real-time examination, although a permanent record of findings can be recorded digitally.

The technique has the advantage of being safe, using non-ionising radiation, being repeatable, painless and requiring little, if any, pre-preparation of the patient. It

Clinical Skills and Examination: The Core Curriculum. By R Turner, B Angus, A Handa, C Hatton. ©2009 Blackwell Publishing, ISBN: 9781405157513.

is also possible to carry out the examination at the patient's bedside and to evaluate a series of organs in a relatively short period of time.

Ultrasound can be used in many different situations, and is used to define the size and texture of internal organs (e.g. hepatomegaly and liver texture; for monitoring of aortic aneurysms), the presence of abnormal masses, and the thickness of the wall of hollow organs (e.g. gallbladder wall/endometrial thickness). Ultrasound is also of use in the detection of gallstones (see Figure 11.1). It may be useful in neonates for imaging the brain, while the anterior fontanelle remains open.

Ultrasound is increasingly used in guiding biopsies of internal organs (e.g. liver biopsy); it may guide pleural aspiration and the placement of central venous catheters.

Radiology

Conventional X-rays visualise only four basic radiographic densities: air, metal, fat and water. Air densities are black; metal densities (the most common of which are calcium and barium) are white with well-defined edges; fat and water densities are dark and mid-grey.

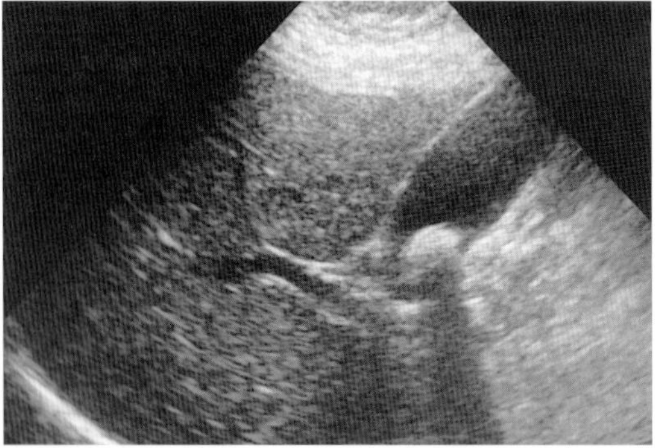

Figure 11.1 Ultrasound scan showing a stone within gallbladder, casting an acoustic shadow.

There can be difficulty in visualising a three-dimensional structure from a two-dimensional film. One helpful rule in deciding where a lesion is situated is to note which, if any, adjacent normal landmarks are obliterated. For example, a water density lesion which obliterates the right border of the heart must lie in the right middle lobe and not the lower lobe. A different view, e.g. lateral chest radiograph, is needed to be certain of the position of densities.

Chest radiograph

Ideally, the chest radiograph should be taken in the posteroanterior (PA) position, to give an accurate representation of heart size. Anteroposterior (AP) radiographs are generally used when the patient is confined to bed. It must be noted that the heart size will appear enlarged (see Figures 11.2 and 11.3).

Abdominal radiography

This is less satisfactory than chest radiography because there are fewer contrasting densities. Air in the gut is

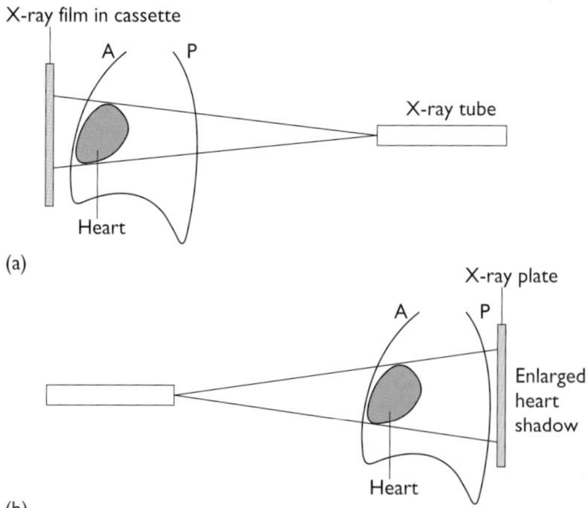

Figure 11.2 (a) A normal posteroanterior (PA) X-ray; (b) an anteroposterior (AP) chest X-ray (mobile X-ray for chest radiographs of patients in bed).

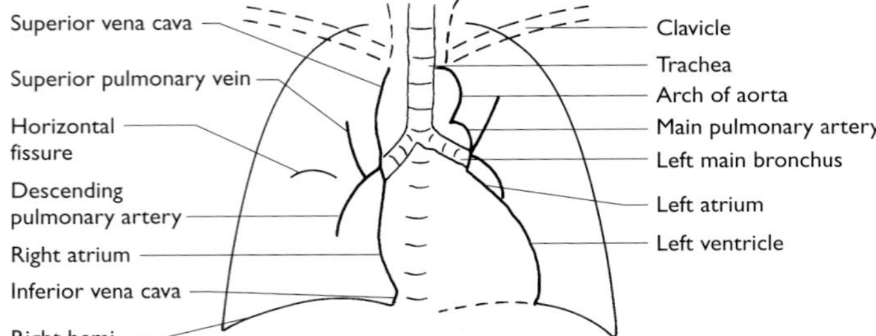

Figure 11.3 Review particularly lungs, apices, costophrenic angles, hilar, behind heart.

helpful, as are the psoas lines. The films are usually taken supine (AP), but an erect radiograph may be taken to define air–fluid levels, suggestive of obstruction.

Barium swallow, meal, enema

Barium is a radio-opaque contrast agent that can outline

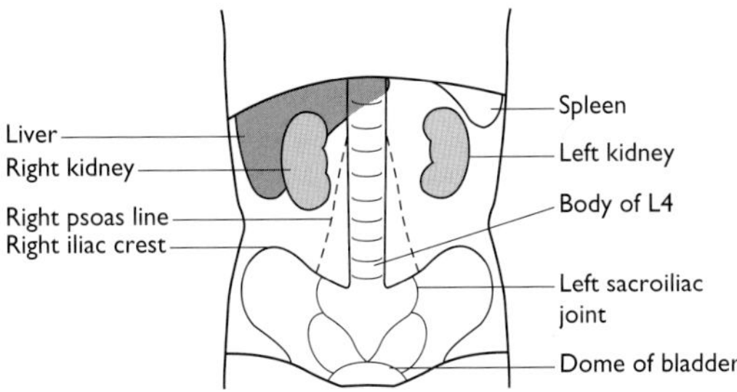

filling defects (e.g. tumours) in the gastrointestinal tract. A barium swallow outlines only the oesophagus; a barium meal is needed to assess the stomach and duodenum. In some cases, a catheter is inserted to introduce barium into the duodenum (small bowel enema). Rectal barium is used to perform a standard barium enema, outlining the large bowel. Interpretation may be complex, with gut contents or peristalsis mimicking filling defects.

Computed tomography (CT)

A segment of the body is X-rayed at numerous angles as the CT apparatus rotates through 360°. A computer summarises the data from multiple pictures to provide a composite image (Figure 11.4). Attenuation of X-rays depends on tissue, and is graded in Hounsfield units. Water is arbitrarily given the value 0, black is –1000 and white is +1000 Hounsfield units. Different 'windows' are chosen to display different characteristics, e.g. soft-tissue window, lung window, bone window.

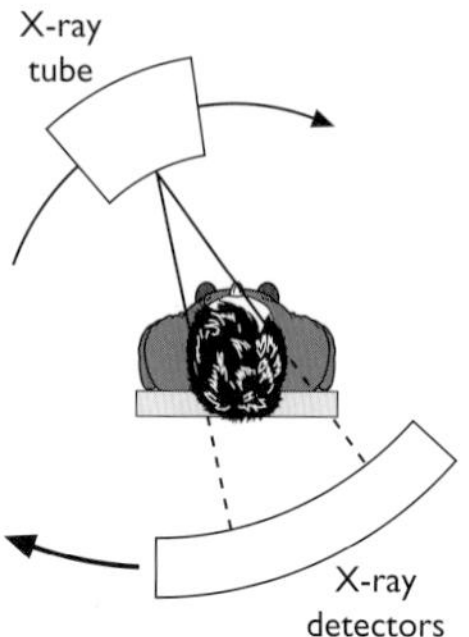

Figure 11.4 Computed tomographic scan across cerebral hemispheres.

The key benefits of CT relate to its better resolution of different body tissues, allowing greater precision in an anatomical localisation.

Variants of CT:

- intravenous contrast
  - iodine-based
  - opacifies blood vessels
  - shows leaky vessels or increased number of vessels—and is therefore useful in demonstrating malignancy
- oral contrast
  - opacifies gut contents
- CTPA—specialised CT technique for demonstrating pulmonary emboli.

Arteriography and venography

An X-ray film is taken after a radiopaque contrast has been injected into a blood vessel (Figure 11.5):

- coronary arteriography, e.g. *coronary artery disease*
- cerebral angiography, e.g. *aneurysm* after *subarachnoid haemorrhage*
- carotid angiography e.g. *stenoses*
- aortography and iliofemoral angiography, e.g. *aortic aneurysm*, *iliofemoral artery atheroma*
- leg venogram, e.g. *deep venous thrombosis*.

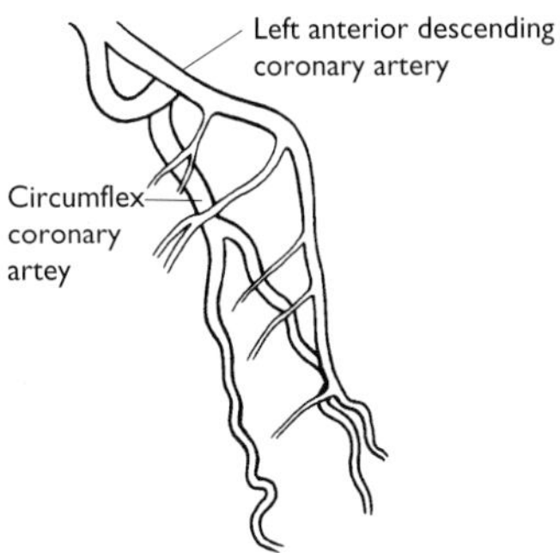

Figure 11.5 Left coronary artery angiogram viewed from right.

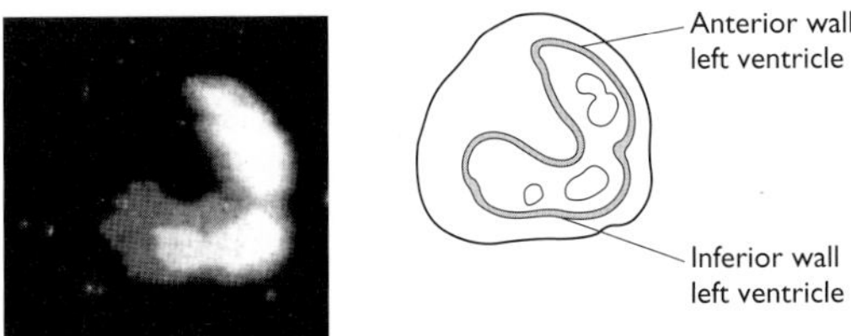

Figure 11.6 Thallium 201 study of the heart.

Concurrent venous blood sampling may help localise an endocrine tumour, e.g. parathormone from an occult parathyroid tumour, catecholamines from a phaeochromocytoma, or to confirm the significance of renal artery stenosis using renal vein renin analyses.

Nuclear medicine studies

These studies use radioactive isotopes (mostly technetium 99 m) coupled to appropriate pharmaceuticals or monoclonal antibodies designed to seek out different organ systems or pathology (Figure 11.6). The studies yield functional rather than morphological information. They are exquisitely sensitive, but not specific.

The following are the commonest investigations routinely available.

Skeletal system

A bone scan may detect any cause of increased bone turnover or altered blood flow to bone, e.g. tumour, infection, trauma, infarction. Used mostly for detection of metastases.

Pulmonary system

Ventilation (V) scan

- Inhalation of an isotope allows picture of parenchyma of the lungs to be taken by a gamma camera.

Perfusion (P) scan

- Injection of isotope into the blood stream demonstrates the blood flow in the lungs.

Mismatch of the scans is used to diagnose pulmonary embolism, i.e. air reaches all parts of the lung, while the blood does not (Figure 11.7). Matching defects occur with other lung pathologies, e.g. *emphysema*.

N.B. A perfusion scan showing an area of ischaemia with a normal chest X-ray is generally sufficient to diagnose a pulmonary embolus. A *V/Q* scan is needed if there is other lung pathology suspected or on X-ray (e.g. chronic bronchitis/emphysema), but in practice the results are difficult to interpret.

Urogenital system

Renography (an activity–time curve of the passage of radioactive tracer through the kidney) for detecting abnormalities of renal blood flow, parenchymal function and excretion. Renal scintigraphy will detect scarring and is used to measure divided renal function. Chromium-51 EDTA (ethylene diamine tetra-acetic acid) clearance measurements yield accurate assessment of glomerular filtration rate.

Thyroid

For estimation of the size, shape and position of the gland, detecting the presence of ‘hot’ thyrotoxic

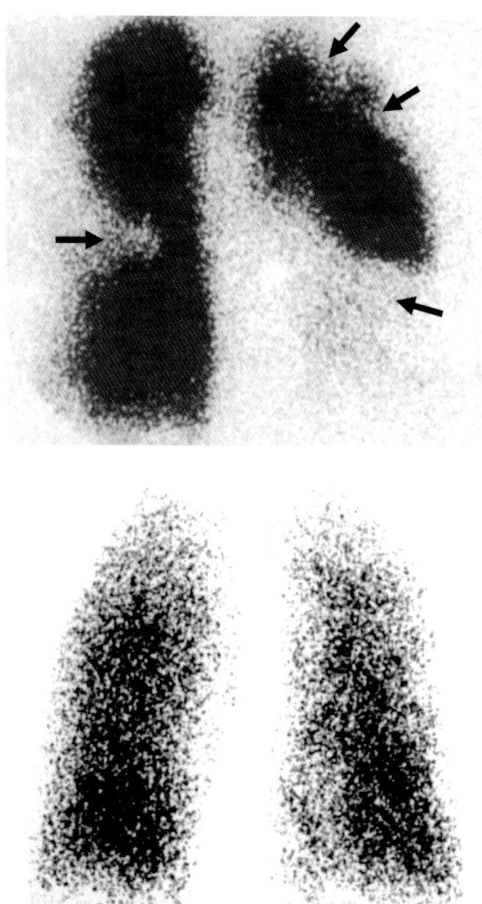

Figure 11.7 V/Q scan of pulmonary embolism: (a) perfusion scan (arrows mark perfusion defects); (b) ventilation scan—normal.

nodules or 'cold' nodules caused by adenoma, carcinoma, cysts, haemorrhage or any combination thereof. Iodine uptake can also be estimated simultaneously.

Adrenals

The detection of autonomously functioning Conn's tumours (cortex) and phaechromocytoma (medulla).

Magnetic resonance imaging

Also known as nuclear magnetic resonance (NMR). Provides cross-sectional images (MRI) or spectroscopic information on chemicals in tissues (magnetic resonance spectroscopy, MRS).

The main strength of MRI is in the imaging of soft tissues and, especially, the central nervous system. It involves no ionising radiation, and is therefore suitable in pregnancy and in children. However, patients with pacemaker and aneurysm clips must not enter the magnet, and any patient with metal implants (e.g. joint replacements) must be discussed with a radiologist.

Gadolinium may be used as a contrast agent in MRI, for example in the detailed imaging of the meninges (Figure 11.8).

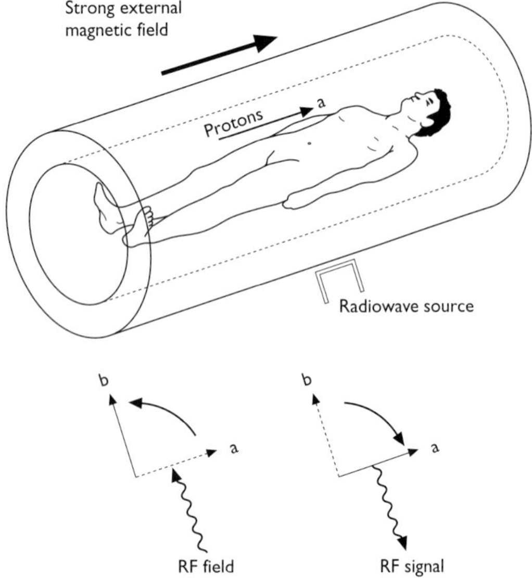

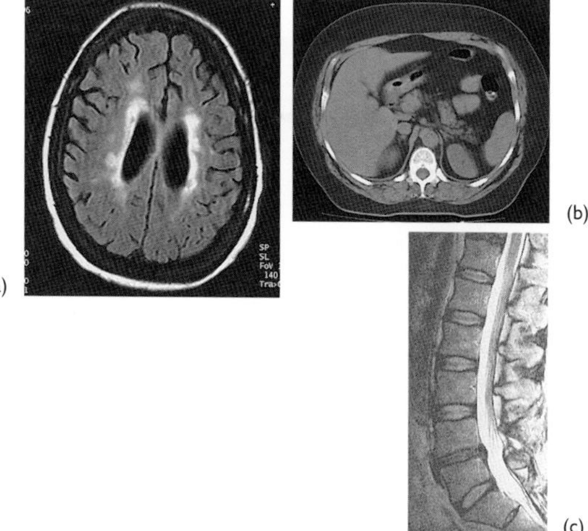

Figure 11.8 (a) MRI T1-weighted scan of the brain. The central white areas are areas of demyelination in multiple sclerosis and subcutaneous fat is white. (b) MRI T2-weighted scan (sagittal section) of the abdomen showing the liver, top of the kidneys, spleen, pancreas, aorta with arterial branches and oral contrast in the jejunum. (c) MRI T2-weighted scan (coronal section) of the lumbar spine showing white central spinal fluid surrounding the spinal cord.

PET scanning

Positron emission tomography (PET) is imaging using 18-F-deoxyglucose (FDG). FDG uptake correlates with glucose metabolism. Malignant tumours actively metabolise glucose, making it possible to image tumours using this technique. PET scanning is useful for identifying malignant deposits which may not be obvious with other conventional imaging techniques. CT-PET allows accurate anatomical localisation of an FDG-avid signal.

Respiratory investigations

pH and arterial blood gases

Normal ranges:

- pH 7.35–7.45
- $P\text{CO}_2$ 4.5–6.2 pK_a
- $P\text{O}_2 > 10.6$ pK_a
- HCO_3^- 22–26 mmol/l
- base excess is the amount of acid required to titrate pH to 7.4

In ventilatory failure:

- $P\text{O}_2$ low
- $P\text{CO}_2$ high

In respiratory failure from lung disease often:

- $P\text{O}_2$ low
- normal $P\text{CO}_2$ due to high carbon dioxide (CO_2) solubility and efficient transfer in lungs.

For example, in asthma, raised CO_2 signifies tiredness and decreased ventilation from reduced muscular effort.

Respiratory acidosis

CO_2 retention from:

- respiratory disease with right-to-left shunt
- ventilatory failure
  - neuromuscular disease
  - physical causes, e.g. flail chest, kyphoscoliosis

Raised CO_2 leads to increased bicarbonate:

$$CO_2 + H_2O = H_2CO_3 = H^+ + HCO_3^-.$$

In chronic respiratory failure, renal compensation by excretion of H^+ and retention of HCO_3^- leads to further increased HCO_3^-, i.e. maintenance of normal pH with compensatory metabolic alkalosis (Figure 11.9).

Respiratory alkalosis

CO_2 blown off by hyperventilation due to:

- hysteria
- brainstem stimulation (rare).

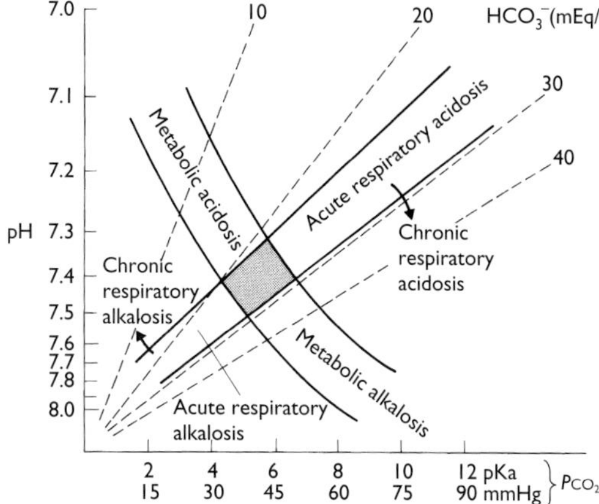

Figure 11.9 Descriptive clinical terms. Shaded area is normal range.

In respiratory alkalosis:

- $P\text{O}_2$ normal
- $P\text{CO}_2$ low.

If chronic, compensated by metabolic acidosis with renal retention of H^+ and excretion of HCO_3^-.

Metabolic acidosis

Excess H^+ in blood:

- ketosis—3-OH butyric acid accumulation in diabetes or starvation
- uraemia—lack of renal H^+ excretion
- renal tubular acidosis—lack of H^+
- acid ingestion—aspirin
- lactic acid accumulation—shock, hypoxia, exercise, metformin
- loss of base—diarrhoea.

Usually compensatory respiratory alkalosis, e.g. Kussmaul respiration of diabetic coma (hyperventilation with deep breathing):

- $P\text{O}_2$ normal
- $P\text{CO}_2$ low.

To assist diagnosis, measure anion gap:

$$[Na^+] + [K^+] - [Cl^-] - [HCO_3^-] = 7 - 16 \text{ mmol/l}.$$

If anion gap >16 mmol/l, unestimated anions are present, e.g. 3-OH butyrate, lactate, formate.

Metabolic alkalosis

Loss of H^+ due to:

- prolonged vomiting
- potassium depletion—secondary to renal tubular potassium–hydrogen exchange
- ingestion of base—old-fashioned sodium bicarbonate therapy of peptic ulcers.

Usually compensatory respiratory acidosis with hypoventilation:

- PO_2 low
- PCO_2 high.

Peak flow

- Blow into machine as hard and fast as you can.
- Records in litres per minute. Useful for diagnosing and observing asthma. Normal range is 300–500 l/min.
- Improvement with β-agonist, e.g. isoprenaline, indicates reversible airway disease, i.e. asthma.

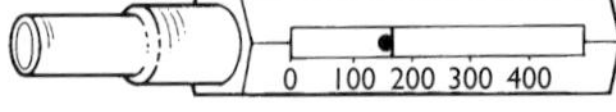

Spirometry

- Blow into machine, a **vitalograph**, as hard as you can—measures pattern of airflow during forced expiration.
- To distinguish between restrictive lung disease, e.g. emphysema, fibrosis and obstructive lung disease, e.g. asthma, chronic obstructive airways disease.

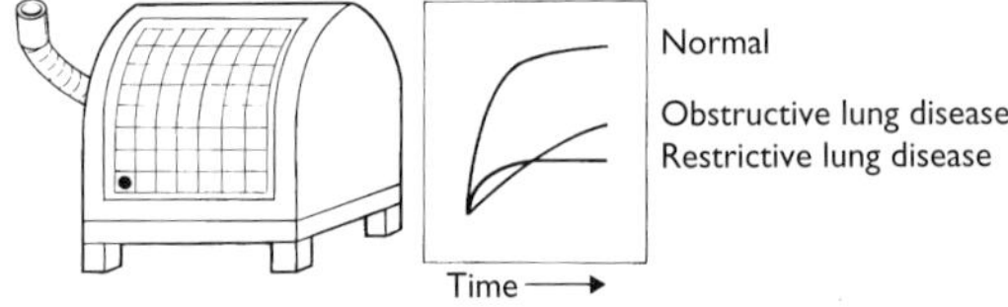

Carbon monoxide transfer factor

The rate of uptake of carbon monoxide from inspired gas determines the lung diffusion capacity. It is reduced in alveolar diseases, e.g. *pulmonary fibrosis*.

Renal investigations

Urine testing

Testing the urine is part of the routine physical examination. It is most simply done using one of the combination dipsticks.

- Dip the stick in the urine and compare the colours with the key at the times specified. Of particular interest are:
  - pH
  - protein content (**N.B.** does not detect Bence Jones protein)
  - ketones
  - glucose
  - bilirubin
  - urobilinogen
  - blood/haemoglobin
  - nitrites.

Urine microscopy

Urine should be sent to the laboratory (sterile) for 'M, C and S':

- M (microscopy)—for the presence of red cells, white cells, casts and pathogens
- C (culture)—using appropriate media to detect bacteria and other pathogens
- S (sensitivity)—to determine the sensitivity of bacteria to antibiotics.

Creatinine clearance

Precise measurements of the **glomerular filtration rate** are made isotopically, e.g. chromium EDTA clearance. The creatinine clearance is easier to organise, although less accurate.

- Collect a blood sample for plasma creatinine.
- Collect a 24-hour urine sample for creatinine.

$$\text{Formula: } \frac{U \times V}{P \times T}:$$

$$\frac{\begin{matrix}\text{Urine creatinine}\\ \text{(mmol)}\end{matrix}}{\begin{matrix}\text{Plasma creatinine}\\ (\mu\text{mol})\end{matrix}} \times \frac{\begin{matrix}\text{Urine volume}\\ (\text{ml}) \times 10^3\end{matrix}}{\begin{matrix}\text{Duration collection}\\ \text{(min)}\end{matrix}} = \begin{matrix}\text{Clearance}\\ \text{(ml/min)}\end{matrix}.$$

Normal value: 80–120 ml/min.

Intravenous urogram

An initial plain film to show renal or ureteric stones. Contrast medium is injected intravenously, concentrated in the kidney and excreted.

- Nephrogram phase—kidneys are outlined
  - observe position, size, shape, filling defects, e.g. tumour.
- Excretion phase—renal pelvis
  - renal papillae may be lost from chronic pyelonephritis, papillary necrosis
  - calyces blunted from hydronephrosis
  - pelviureteric obstruction—large pelvis, normal ureters.
- Ureters—observe position—displaced by other pathology?
  - size—dilated from obstruction or recent infection
  - irregularities—may be contractions and need to be checked in sequential films.

CT urograms have largely superseded this investigation in some centres.

Neurological investigations

Electroencephalogram

Approximately 22 electrodes are applied to the scalp in standard positions and cerebral electrical activity is amplified and recorded. There are marked normal variations and differences between awake and sleep.

Main uses

- Epilepsy
  - primary, generalised epilepsy—generalised spike and slow-wave discharges
  - partial epilepsy—focal spikes
- Disorders of consciousness or coma
  - encephalopathy
  - encephalitis
  - dementia

The main value of this technique is in showing episodes of abnormal waves compatible with epilepsy. Large normal variation makes interpretation difficult.

Lumbar puncture

A needle is introduced between the lumbar vertebrae (Figure 11.10), through the dura into the subarachnoid space, and cerebrospinal fluid is obtained for examination.

Normal cerebrospinal fluid is completely clear.

The major diagnostic value of this technique is in:

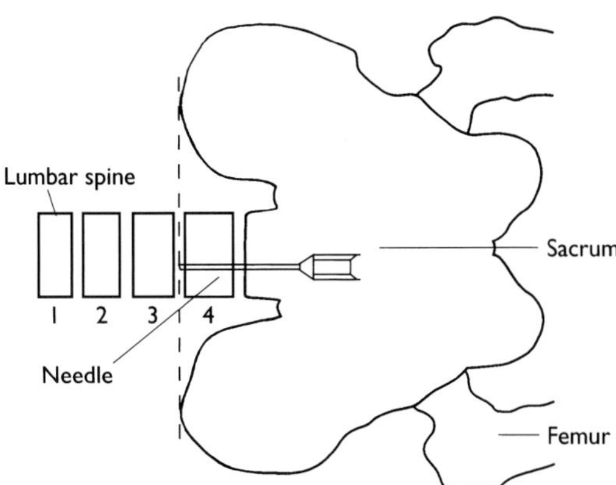

Figure 11.10 The lumbar puncture needle is positioned between L3 and L4 to one side of the supraspinous ligament.

- subarachnoid haemorrhage—uniformly red, whereas blood from a 'traumatic' tap is in the first specimen
  - xanthochromia—yellow stain from haemoglobin breakdown
- meningitis—pyogenic, turbid fluid, white cells, organisms on culture, low glucose and raised protein
- raised pressure may indicate a tumour.

Haematological investigations

Full blood count and film examination

Blood should be taken into EDTA anticoagulant (purple-topped vacutainer) from venous puncture for analysis by automated cell counters. Most laboratories will be able to deliver the following parameters.

Hb (g/l or g/dl)	concentration of haemoglobin and the indicator of anaemia
RBC	red cell count, expressed as a number per litre
MCV (fl)	the mean cell volume; is useful in determining the cause of anaemia—microcytic (<76fl), normocytic or macrocytic (>96fl)
MCH (pg)	mean corpuscular haemoglobin measured in picograms; this defines hypochromia when <27 pg
MCHC	mean corpuscular haemoglobin concentration; not generally useful
WBC	total white cell count expressed as a number $\times 10^9$/l
Platelets	total platelet count expressed as a number $\times 10^9$/l

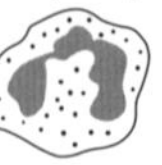

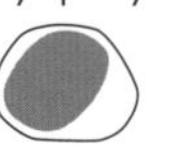

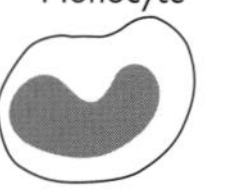

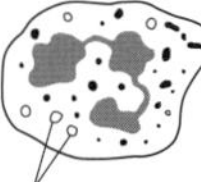

Most automated blood analysers will provide a five-part differential white cell count, thereby defining by percentage and absolute number of neutrophils, lymphocytes, monocytes, eosinophils and basophils present.

Blood film examination provides additional morphological information of blood cells and should always be requested in anaemia of unknown cause, abnormalities of white cell or platelet counts.

Red cells

Anaemia results from a reduction in the haemoglobin concentration—the causes of which include:

- bleeding
- haemolysis (premature destruction of red cells)—high reticulocyte count
- bone marrow disease (failure of production)
- haematinic deficiency (B_{12}, folate, iron)
- renal failure (reduction of erythropoietin)
- chronic inflammation and malignancy

The **MCV** is an indicator of the cause of anaemia:

- **microcytic**—Fe deficiency, thalassaemia trait
- **macrocytic**—B_{12} or folate deficiency, hypothyroidism, liver disease, alcohol abuse and bone marrow disease
- **normochromic**—chronic disease, renal failure and malignancy.

Inspection of the **blood film** can provide useful information regarding the aetiology of anaemia. Red cell morphology is important in identifying causes of haemolysis, e.g. spherocytes, fragmented cells, sickle cells.

Haemoglobin electrophoresis. Electrophoresis of a red cell lysate will identify haemoglobin variants such as haemoglobin S-HbS. The detection and measurement of HbA_2 is very important for the detection of carriers of thalassaemia. HbA_2 >3.5% is suggestive of β-thalassaemia trait carrier status.

Red cell enzymes. Deficiency of red cell enzymes such as G6PD and PK can lead to a severe haemolytic anaemia. Such enzymes can be assayed in the laboratory.

White cells

An abnormal white cell count needs attention. Blood film examination may identify the presence of abnormal cells such as blasts, or may simply show an elevation or reduction of normal components. The presence of abnormal white cell morphology may be an indication for a bone marrow biopsy.

- **Neutrophilia**—elevated neutrophil count; usually indicative of bacterial infection.
- **Neutropenia**—a low neutrophil count can lead to serious infection (Gram-negative sepsis) often related to chemotherapy but temporarily may follow simple viral infection.
- **Lymphocytosis**—reactive in viral infections such as glandular fever; clonal in lymphoid leukaemias and lymphoma.
- **Lymphopenia**—common in patients taking steroids, human immunodeficiency virus (HIV), systemic lupus erythematosus (SLE) and other autoimmune disease.
- **Eosinophilia**—common in atopy and allergic states. Occurs in association with drugs, parasitic infection and lymphoma.

Coagulation

Blood should be taken into citrate (light blue-topped vacutainer tube). Citrate reversibly binds Ca^{2+} and prevents the sample from clotting. In the laboratory the blood is centrifuged and the plasma removed for testing. A source of tissue factor/phospholipid (thromboplastin) is added and Ca^{2+} added. The time to clot in seconds is measured.

- **Prothrombin time (PT)** (normally 10–14 seconds) is a measure of the extrinsic (tissue factor/VII dependent) system. It is very sensitive to vitamin K-dependent factors (II, VII, IX and X).

- The PT is the most sensitive **liver function test**—prolonged in liver disease.
- The PT is the most sensitive clotting test with which to **monitor warfarin therapy**—warfarin inhibits vitamin K-dependent clotting factors (II, VII, IX and X). The PT of the patient/PT of pooled normal plasma gives a ratio—the prothrombin ratio. If the PT ratio is multiplied by a correction for the 'sensitivity' of the thromboplastin used (international sensitivity ratio, ISI) the **INR** or **international normalised ratio** is derived.

Target INR	Clinical condition
2.0–3.0	Treatment of deep venous thrombosis (DVT) or pulmonary embolism (PE)
3.0–4.5	Anticoagulation for prosthetic valves and grafts; treatment of thromboembolism occurring on warfarin

- Activated partial thromboplastin time (APTT)—this measures the so-called intrinsic system. This pathway is slower and requires both phospholipid and a surface activator (e.g. kaolin—as in the kaolin cephalin thromboplastin time, KCTT). Patients' plasma from citrated blood is added to a source of phospholipid, kaolin and Ca^{2+}. The time to clot is measured and is usually in the order of 30–40 seconds). The test is used for:
  - Monitoring heparin when the APTT is usually kept at about 2.5 × normal. **N.B.** low molecular weight heparin usually does not require monitoring with the exception of renal failure when a factor Xa assay is performed.
  - This test is prolonged in the presence of the antiphospholipid antibody.
  - The test is prolonged in haemophilia and von Willebrand's disease.

- **Other coagulation tests include the thrombin time (TT)**, which is sensitive to heparin therapy, and the **fibrinogen level**, which is a direct measurement of the fibrinogen concentration of the blood. Disseminated intravascular coagulation usually causes a prolongation of all the above coagulation tests and a reduction in the level of fibrinogen.
- **D-dimers**—activation of the fibrinolytic system follows the formation of a clot. Plasmin becomes activated and cleaves the polymerised fibrin into smaller molecules (some of which are called D-dimers). D-dimers can be detected using either a latex agglutination or an ELISA-based test. The detection of D-dimers may infer the presence of clot and is now used in the diagnosis of DVT and PE; while very sensitive, it is not specific, however. Absence of D-dimers implies absence of significant thrombosis.
- **Thrombophilia tests**—a number of components of the blood help prevent the formation of spontaneous blood clots. These factors work by interrupting the coagulation cascade. Deficiencies can make patients susceptible to thrombosis. Most of these factor deficiencies are inherited—**taking a family history is very important**. The most common inherited thrombophilic defect is Factor V Leiden, but numerous acquired features may also contribute to the risk of thromboembolism.

Cross-matching blood for transfusion

Before blood can be safely administered to a patient, the patient's serum must be screened for red cell antibodies that may cause a transfusion reaction should the corresponding antigen be present on the donor red cells. A sample of blood (varies in different laboratories—clot or EDTA) must be sent to the transfusion laboratory before blood can be issued. Careful labelling/identification of all samples is essential. The laboratory process involves:

- ABO and RhD blood grouping
- serum/plasma from the patient is reacted with donor red cells
- once the ABO and RhD blood group has been determined and the absence of red cell antibodies has been confirmed, blood can be issued.

Emergency blood for transfusion

There are rare occasions when there is insufficient time to allow for cross-matching. In this situation group O Rh-neg emergency stock can be given. (Must liaise directly with transfusion laboratory.)

Special requirements

Certain patients have special transfusion requirements—some of these are listed here:

- **irradiated blood product**—patients will carry a card
- **cytomegalovirus (CMV)-negative blood products** may be required in:
  - patients undergoing organ transplantation
  - neonates.

Bone marrow biopsy

This biopsy is usually taken from the iliac crest (most often posterior) and is performed in two parts.

1. The aspirate is marrow that is sucked out of the marrow cavity and spread on a glass slide, stained and examined under a microscope to determine cellular morphology. The sample may also be stained with Perl's Prussian blue stain, which will give the best indication as to the patient's iron status.
2. The trephine involves taking a bone marrow core, which is fixed in formalin, decalcified and then sectioned in the normal histological manner. The trephine will identify bone marrow infiltration with secondary carcinoma, fibrosis, haematological malignancies and best defines the cellularity of the marrow.

The procedure is either carried out with simple infiltration of the periosteum using local anaesthetic or under light sedation.

Biochemical tests

- **Urea and electrolytes**—measurement of sodium, potassium, urea and creatinine. Urea is useful in assessment of dehydration. It is dependent on protein loads—elevated by high protein meals or gastrointestinal bleeds, reduced by liver dysfunction. **Creatinine** is the most reliable simple test of glomerular function.
- **Anion gap**—difference in the sum of principal cations (sodium and potassium) and anions (chloride and bicarbonate) = 14–18 mmol/l (represents unmeasured negative charge on plasma proteins). Useful in investigation of acid–base alterations.
- **Liver functions tests**—better described as **liver profile** as the tests do not really reflect liver function.
  - **Albumin**—mainly responsible for maintaining colloid osmotic pressure and a useful marker of liver synthetic function. May be dramatically reduced in nephrotic syndrome and protein-losing enteropathy.
  - **AST and ALT** (aspartate transaminase and alanine amino transferase)—these enzymes are released in liver damage, but also present in red cells, muscle and cardiac cells. May be very high in hepatitis.
  - **Bilirubin**—breakdown product of haemoglobin and therefore elevated in haemolysis. Also elevated in liver disease.
  - **ALP** (alkaline phosphatase)—an enzyme found in osteoblasts and the hepatobiliary system. Elevated in bone disease and biliary obstruction.
  - **GGT** (gamma glutamyl-transferase)—increased in alcohol abuse.
  - **Amylase** enzyme produced by the pancreas for digestion of complex carbohydrates. Elevated in pancreatitis.

- **Cardiac/muscle markers**
  - **Troponins (T and I)**—most specific and sensitive markers of myocardial damage, rising early after myocardial injury. A rise in troponin defines the acute coronary syndrome. Older tests such as CK MB and AST/LDH are now largely obsolete in this setting
- **Calcium/bone metabolism**
  - Most abundant mineral in the body, though 99% is bound within bone. Plasma levels need adjusting for the albumin concentration before interpretation.

Adjusted calcium =

$$(40 - (\text{albumin concentration } (g/l))) \times 0.02 \text{ mmol/l}$$

- Homeostasis of calcium is affected by parathyroid hormone (PTH) (↑) and vitamin D action.
  - **Phosphate**—most commonly elevated in renal insufficiency. Very high levels are found in tumour lysis. Plasma levels affected by PTH and vitamin D action.
  - **PTH**—released from parathyroid glands in response to a reduction in calcium and results in increased renal tubular absorption of calcium and increased phosphate excretion. Also releases calcium and phosphate from bone and leads to renal activation of vitamin D.
  - **Vitamin D**—activated by hydroxylation in liver and kidney. Stimulates increased absorption of calcium and phosphate from the gut. Increases osteoblast bone resorption.
- **Lipid profile (take samples fasting)**
  - **Cholesterol**—important membrane structural component. Precursor of all steroid and bile acid synthesis. Elevated levels correlated with increased risk of cardiovascular disease, especially if LDL is elevated.
  - **LDL (low density lipoprotein)**—principal carrier of cholesterol, attaching to LDL cell surface receptors to allow internalisation. Independent cardiovascular risk factor.

- **HDL (high density lipoprotein)**—functions to reverse cholesterol transport, carrying cholesterol back to the liver for metabolism, therefore, cardioprotective.
- **Triglycerides**—present in dietary fat and synthesised by liver to provide store of energy. Independent cardiovascular risk factor. Elevated in liver disease and hypothyroidism.

Endocrinology

Anterior pituitary hormones

- **TSH (thryoid stimulating hormone)**—stimulates production of thyroxine (T4) and tri-iodothyronine (T3) from the thyroid gland. Diagnosis of hypo- or hyperthyroidism depends on TSH measurement.
- **ACTH (adrenocorticotrophic hormone)**—increases cortisol production from the adrenal glands in response to stress, daily variation, infection, etc.
  - Cortisol excess is known as Cushing's syndrome or Cushing's disease (pituitary-driven ACTH).
  - Cortisol deficiency from adrenal failure is known as Addison's disease.
- **GH (growth hormone)**—stimulates growth in pre-pubertal children and has many diffuse effects on adult metabolism. GH is activated by insulin-like growth factor 1 (IGF-1) in the liver. An excess of growth hormone in adulthood produces acromegaly.
- **Prolactin**—milk gland-stimulating hormone elevated in pregnancy and lactation. Very high levels in some pituitary adenomata.
- **FSH (follicle stimulating hormone)**—gonadotrophin which nurtures the development of the follicle in the first half of the menstrual cycle. In males FSH stimulates spermatogenesis. High levels are found in post-menopausal women.
- **LH (luteinising hormone)**—elevated in the second half of the menstrual cycle producing development of the corpus luteum. In males LH stimulates testosterone synthesis.

Table 11.1 Diagnosis of glycaemic status.

Diagnosis	Timing	Plasma glucose (mmol/l)
Physiological	Fasting	<6.1
Impaired fasting glucose	Fasting	>6.1 <7.0
	2-hour OGTT	<7.8
Impaired glucose tolerance	Fasting	<7.0
	2-hour OGTT	>7.8 <11.1
Diabetes mellitus	Fasting	>7.0
	2-hour OGTT	>11.1

Posterior pituitary hormone

- **ADH (antidireutic hormone)**—decreases water loss. Absence of ADH causes diabetes insipidus. Conditions that cause inappropriate ADH secretion (various tumours) lead to a fall in plasma sodium. Measurement of **urine and plasma osmolarity**.

Dynamic endocrine tests

- **Short Synacthen test**—injection of synthetic ACTH at time 0 after blood sampling. Further blood samples are taken at 30 and 60 minutes. A physiological response results in an elevation of cortisol peak to >570 nmol/l. A reduced response is seen in Addison's disease (adrenal failure).
- **Oral glucose tolerance test (OGTT)**—used to diagnose diabetes mellitus by demonstrating abnormal glucose handling (Table 11.1).
- **Insulin tolerance test**—used to demonstrate the normal reactivity of cortisol and growth hormone (both antagonise the action of insulin) to hypoglycaemia induced by insulin. Abnormal response seen in adrenal failure or growth hormone deficiency.
- **Testing for Cushing's syndrome**
  - **Outpatient screening test**
  - ***1 mg overnight dexamethasone suppression test***—1 mg of dexamethasone is administered at 11.00 pm or midnight; clotted or lithium heparin sample

for cortisol measurement is taken at 8.00–9.00 am (supraphysiological steroid dose should suppress endogenous production when cortisol is sampled next morning).

- ***Urinary cortisol output***—24-hour urine collection to measure urinary free cortisol.
- **Inpatient screening tests—liaise with endocrinologists.** Involves low and high dose dexamethasone suppression tests, midnight cortisol sampling and radiological examination of the pituitary, adrenals and any other relevant ectopic source.

Immunological investigations

- **Antinuclear antibody**—Can be of any immunoglobulin (Ig) class. Staining pattern is associated with specific diseases.

Homogeneous	lupus
Speckled	mixed connective tissue disease
Nucleolar staining	scleroderma
Centromere staining	CREST syndrome (calcinosis, Raynaud's phenomenon, oesophageal motility abnormalities, scleroderma and telangiectasia)

- **Antismooth muscle antibody**—elevated in autoimmune hepatitis.
- **Gastric parietal cell**—seen in patients with pernicious anaemia (90%).
- **Intrinsic factor antibodies**—70% of pernicious anaemia patients; more specific.
- **Mitochondrial antibody**—96% of patients with primary biliary cirrhosis.
- **Anti-endomysial and antigliadin antibodies**—coeliac disease.
- **Thyroid antibody**—antithyroglobulin elevated in autoimmune thyroiditis (90%); antimicrosomal antibody elevations may be seen in Grave's disease.

- **Rheumatoid factor**—antibody against human IgG but can be of any Ig class. Positive in 70% of rheumatoid arthritis, particularly extra-articular involvement. Very high levels in cryoglobulinaemia.
- **ANCA (antineutrophil cytoplasmic antibodies)**
  - **Cytoplasmic ANCA (cANCA)**—90% of Wegener's granulomatosis; 40% of patients with microscopic polyangiitis.
  - **Perinuclear ANCA (pANCA)**—60% of microscopic polyangiitis patients; may also be positive in connective tissue disorders and vasculitic diseases.
  - After applying blood to the strip, the result is shown after about 20 seconds.

CHAPTER 12
Endoscopy

Introduction

In endoscopy, internal organs, a hollow viscus or an anatomical space are directly visualised, usually with a flexible fibreoptic endoscope.

Oesophago-gastroduodenoscopy (OGD)

A flexible scope is inserted by mouth, after intravenous diazepam, for direct vision of the oesophagus, stomach and duodenum.

It is usually undertaken as a day case, and common indications are reflux symptoms, peptic ulcer disease, dysphagia or suspected upper gastro-intestinal bleeding.

It is now the first line investigation of the upper GI tract as it allows direct visualisation, biopsy for tissue diagnosis as well as therapeutic manoeuvres (**e.g. injection for bleeding, dilatation of strictures**). (See also Upper GI endoscopy.)

Proctoscopy

With the patient lying in a left lateral position on one side, with knees and hips flexed, a short tube is introduced through the anus with a removable obturator lubricated with gel. A light attachment then allows visualisation of the anus and part of the rectum. It is usually used to investigate **rectal bleeding**—haemorrhoids, fistula or anal carcinoma. Haemorrhoids can be injected with phenol or banded with rubber bands to stop bleeding as an outpatient procedure.

Clinical Skills and Examination: The Core Curriculum. By R Turner, B Angus, A Handa, C Hatton. ©2009 Blackwell Publishing, ISBN: 9781405157513.

Sigmoidoscopy (rigid or flexible)

With the patient in left lateral position, either a rigid tube with a removable obturator or a flexible fibreoptic endoscope is introduced. The bowel is kept patent with air from a hand pump. Patients for a flexible sigmoidoscopy usually need an enema to empty the whole of the left side of the colon and allow visualisation of the rectum, and the sigmoid as well as the descending colon. It can be undertaken as an outpatient procedure in the clinic setting. Usually used to investigate:

- **bleeding, diarrhoea or constipation (change in bowel habit)**—*ulcerative colitis*, other *inflammatory bowel disease* or *carcinoma*
- **inflamed area or lumps can be biopsied.**

Colonoscopy

After the bowel is emptied with an oral purgative and a washout if necessary, the whole of the colon and possibly the terminal ileum can be examined. Allows a biopsy to be undertaken and also treatment of polyps by diathermy excision. Usually undertaken as a day case and used to investigate:

- **bleeding, diarrhoea or constipation, change in bowel habit or tenesmus**—*inflammatory bowel disease*, *polyps* or *carcinoma*.

Bronchoscopy

After intravenous diazepam, the major bronchi are observed. Usually undertaken as a day case and also allows biopsy as well as excision with diathermy or laser cauterisation of lesions. It is used to investigate:

- **haemoptysis or suspected bronchial obstruction**—*bronchial carcinoma* and for clearing *obstructed bronchi*, e.g. peanuts, plug of mucus. May also be used for bronchial lavage washings to make a diagnosis of lung infections or tumour.

Laparoscopy

After general anaesthetic, organs can be observed through a small abdominal incision, aspirated for cells or organisms, or biopsied. Laparoscopic surgery includes sterilisation, ova collection for *in vitro* fertilisation and laparoscopic cholecystectomy. Increasingly, laparoscopic techniques are being used for adrenal, colonic, renal, gastric and also vascular surgery. This is a rapidly developing area of surgery. Most surgeons are training to undertake some of their practice laparoscopically.

Cystoscopy

After local anaesthetic, a cystoscope is inserted into the urethral meatus and then into the bladder. Check cystoscopies are mostly undertaken in the outpatient setting and therapeutic resections of bladder tumours as day cases. It allows tissue biopsies as well as therapeutic manoeuvres. It is used to investigate:

- **urinary bleeding or poor flow**—*bladder tumours*
- under direct vision, catheters can be inserted into ureters for retrograde pyelograms and the treatment of ureteric calculi.

Colposcopy

Examination of the cervix, usually to take a cervical smear. Undertaken as an outpatient and can also allow cone biopsy of the cervix. It is used to investigate:

- **premalignant changes or cancer.**

Upper gastrointestinal endoscopy

A flexible fibreoptic tube is introduced into the oesophagus, stomach and duodenum after mild sedation, e.g. intravenous diazepam, with local anaesthetic to pharynx.

It allows direct vision of the gastrointestinal tract to investigate:

- **dysphagia**—oesophageal tumour or stricture
- **haematemesis or melaena**—oesophageal varices, gastric and duodenal ulcers, superficial gastric erosions, gastric carcinoma

- **epigastric pain**—peptic ulcer, oesophagitis, gastritis, duodenitis
- **unexplained weight loss**—gastric carcinoma.

Endoscopic retrograde cholangiopancreatography (ERCP)
Through a fibreoptic endoscope, with a picture on a video, under direct vision, a tube is inserted through the ampulla of Vater at the opening of the common bile duct, and introduction of a radio-paque contrast medium allows X-ray visualisation of:

- **biliary tree**, for stones, tumours, strictures, irregularities
- **pancreatic ducts**, for chronic pancreatitis, dilated ducts or distortion from a tumour.

The endoscope can be used for surgery, including **sphincterotomy** of ampulla for removal of gallstones in the bile duct or the introduction of a rigid tube, **a stent**, through a constricting tumour to allow biliary drainage.

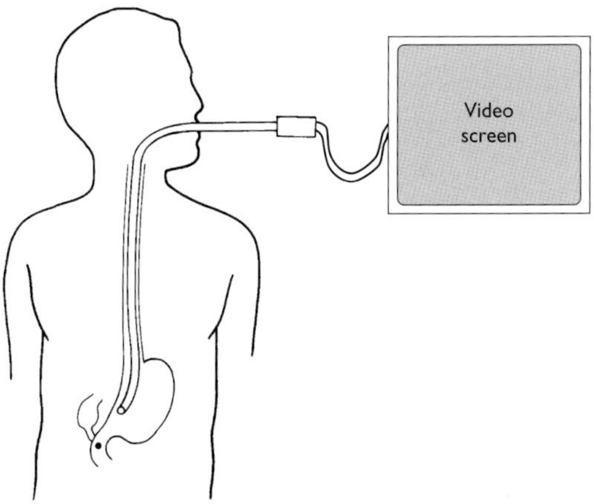

Consent

This should be undertaken for all interactions with patients, even history taking. Always introduce yourself, state your designation (e.g. I am a medical student) and then explicitly ask for consent (permission) to take a history and to examine the patient.

This is particularly important for intimate examinations and you should NOT undertake these without a chaperone present. Always try to maintain as much dignity as possible in your examination so that you are not leaving the patient exposed unnecessarily. There is a balance between adequate exposure to allow adequate examination and over-exposure.

Examinations

Explain to the patient what you are going to do and why it is necessary, e.g. rectal examination or proctoscopy. Make sure they understand what you are going to do and give them an opportunity to ask questions before you start. After the examination/procedure, let them get dressed behind a curtain before discussing the findings. As a general rule, try not to talk to patients until they are dressed or covered up and sitting on a chair or sitting up in bed.

Procedures/Operations

Consent should be undertaken by someone who is either capable of performing the procedure OR has been trained to take consent for that procedure.

Try to use the following guidelines.

- Find a quiet place to talk (or draw the curtains if an in-patient).
- Confirm their name and date of birth to ensure you have the correct patient.
- Explain what the procedure/operation planned is in simple plain language.
- Explain what the intended benefits of the procedure are.
- Explain what the common risks of the procedure are (you should discuss any risks with a greater than 1% incidence or those that have a high morbidity).
- Give the patient an information leaflet if available.

- Give them some idea of the recovery from the procedure.
- Give them an opportunity to ask any questions.
- In general, ask them if they would like a family member or friend to be present.
- Give them a copy of the consent form.

As a student, take the time to watch others take consent. Think about how you would feel if you were the patient. Then pick up aspects of good practice or phrases that you think worked well and do not use aspects that you thought were sub-optimal.

Remember, practice makes perfect, and try to watch as many people taking consent as possible and then practise yourself with colleagues or your teachers watching.

CHAPTER 13
Cardiological investigations

Electrocardiogram

The 12-lead electrocardiogram (ECG) tracings arise from the electrical changes, depolarisation and repolarisation that accompany muscle contraction. With knowledge of the relative position of the leads to the electrodes, the ECG tracings provide direct information of the cardiac muscle and its activity.

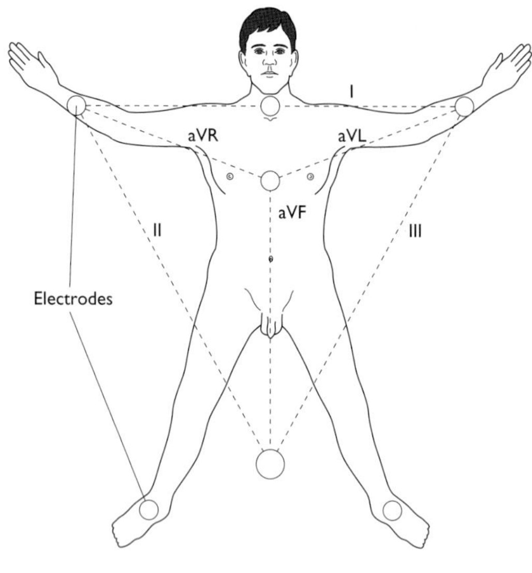

Clinical Skills and Examination: The Core Curriculum. By R Turner, B Angus, A Handa, C Hatton. ©2009 Blackwell Publishing, ISBN: 9781405157513.

Six **standard leads**—I, II, III, aVR, aVL, aVF—are recorded from the limb electrodes (aV = augmented voltage) and examine the heart from different directions.

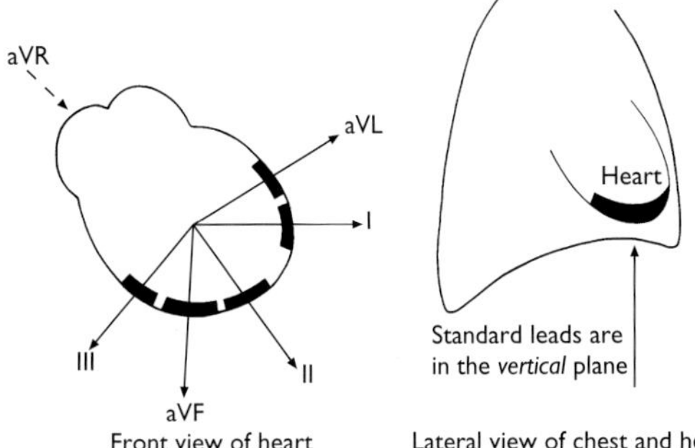

Front view of heart

Lateral view of chest and heart

The standard leads examine the heart in the **vertical** plane.

Six chest leads, V leads, attached by sticky electrodes to the chest wall, are all in the **horizontal** plane.

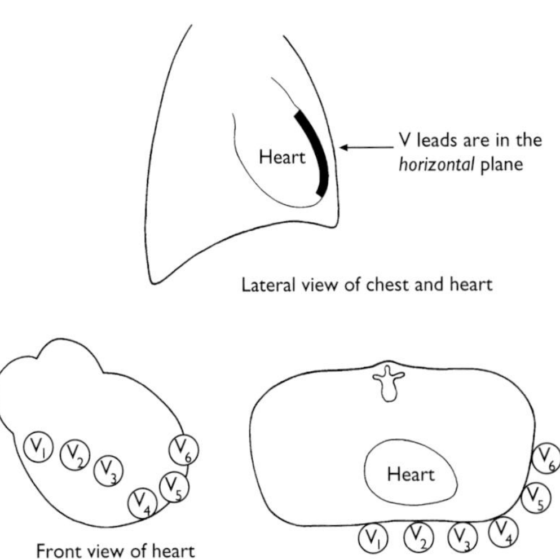

Front view of heart

Obstruction of arteries gives appropriate specific patterns of ischaemia:

- left anterior descending coronary artery—*anterior ischaemia* or *infarct* (V_{1-6})
- circumflex coronary artery—*lateral ischaemia* or *infarct* (I, aVL)
- right coronary artery—*inferior ischaemia* or *infarct* (II, III, aVF)

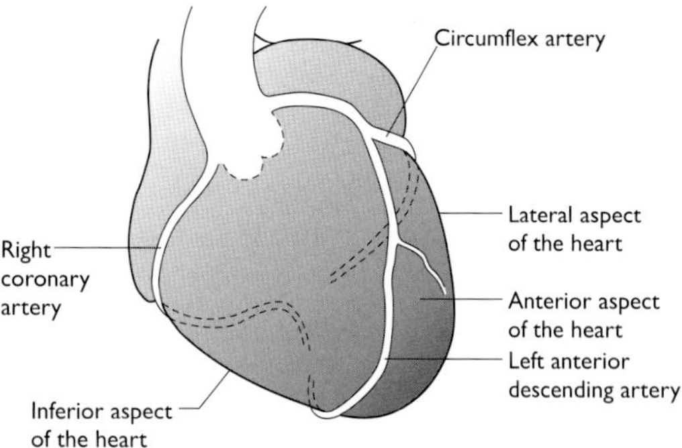

Every ECG tracing must first be standardised by making sure the 1 mV mark deviates the pointer 10 small squares on the paper.

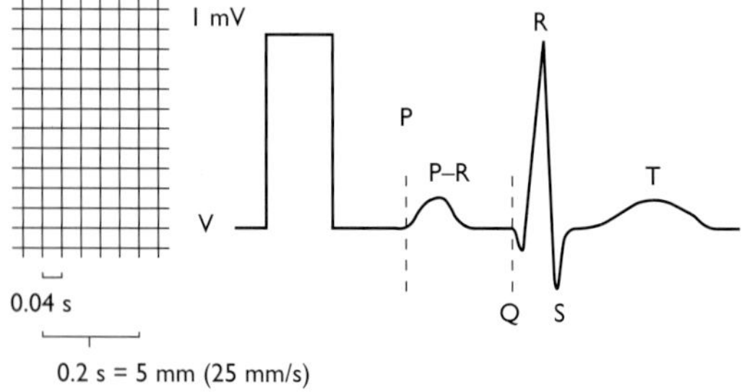

P = atrial depolarisation, QRS = ventricular depolarisation, T = repolarisation.

Normal ECG

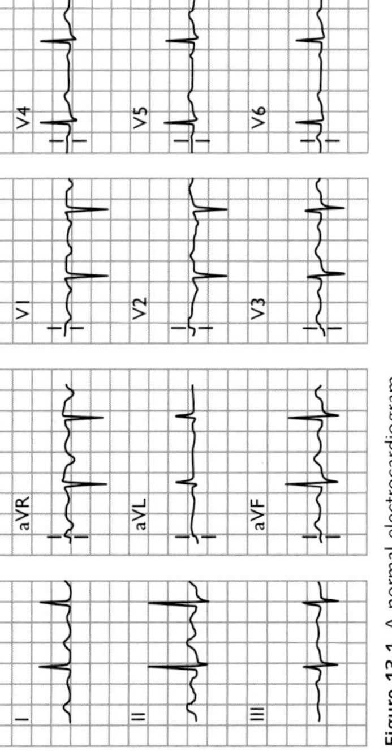

Figure 13.1 A normal electrocardiogram.

Normal ECG variants

- T waves can be inverted in leads III, aVF, V_{1-3}.
- T waves and P waves are always inverted in aVR (if not, leads are misplaced).
- In a young athletic person:
  - ST segments may be raised, especially in leads V_{1-5}
  - right bundle-branch block (RBBB) may occur
  - electrical criteria of left ventricular hypertrophy may be present
  - bradycardia <40 beats/min
  - physiological Q waves.
- Ectopics of any type, including ventricular, are rarely of significance.
- Raised ST segments are common in Afro-Caribbean subjects.
- P mitrale is overdiagnosed:
  - P wave in V_1 is often biphasic.

Electrophysiology of cardiac contractions

All cardiac muscle has a tendency to depolarisation, leading to excitation and contraction.

Initial electrical discharge from the sinoatrial (SA) node (under influence of sympathetic and parasympathetic control) spreads to the atrioventricular (AV) node and via the bundle of His to the ventricles.

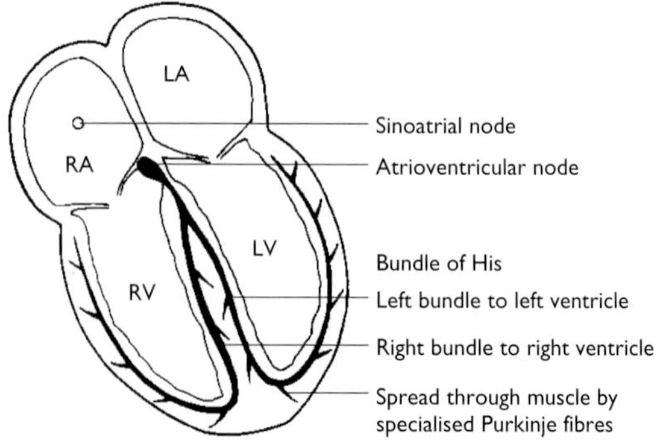

The deflection of the ECG tracing indicates the average direction of all muscle activity at each moment.

Depolarisation spreads:

- towards lead—ECG tracing moves up the paper
- away from lead—tracing moves down paper.

P wave

- depolarisation spreads from SA node to AV node through the atrial muscle fibres (1 in figure below)
- best seen in leads II and V_1
- usually small, as atria are small.

Normal P wave <2.5 mm high, <2.5 mm wide.

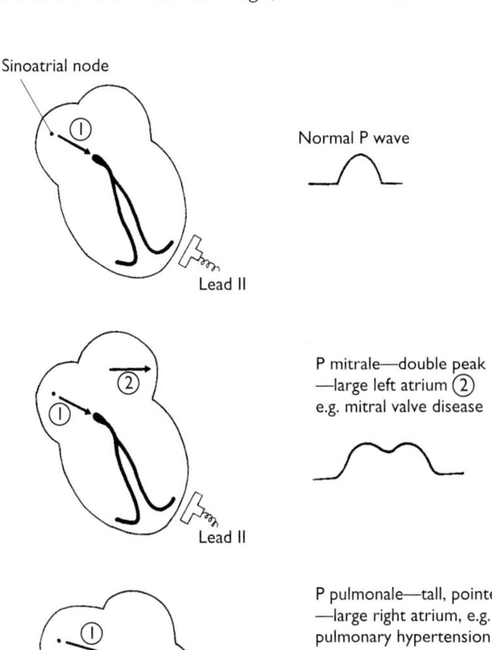

QRS complex

The QRS deflections have a standard nomenclature:

Q—any initial deflection downwards.

R—any deflection upwards, whether or not a preceding Q.

S—any deflection downwards after an R wave, whether or not a preceding Q.

Q

R or R Q

R S or R Q S

QRS in the V leads

RV LV V_1 V_2 V_3 V_4 V_5 V_6

Usually: V_{1-2} opposite R ventricle

V_{3-4} opposite septum

V_{5-6} opposite L ventricle

The septum depolarises first from left to right.

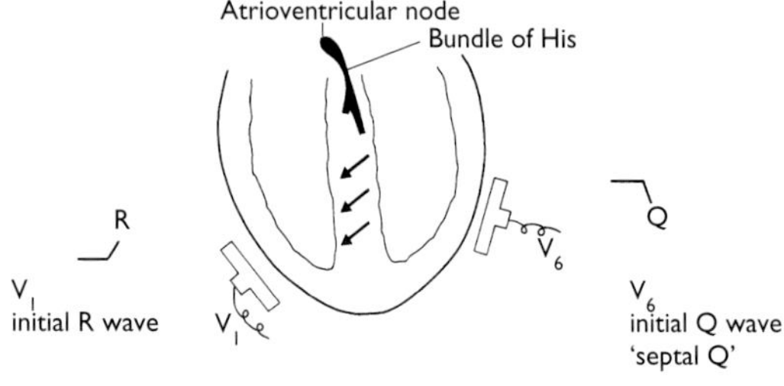

The ventricles then depolarise from inside outwards. The large left ventricle then normally dominates.

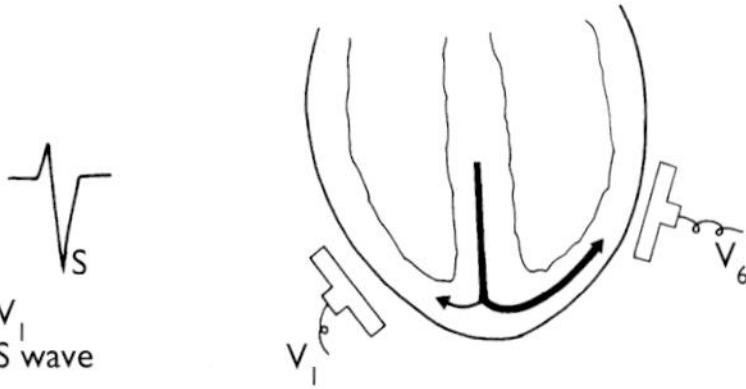

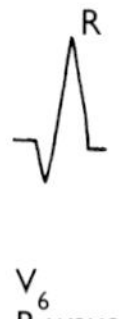

The transition point where R and S are equal is the position of the septum.

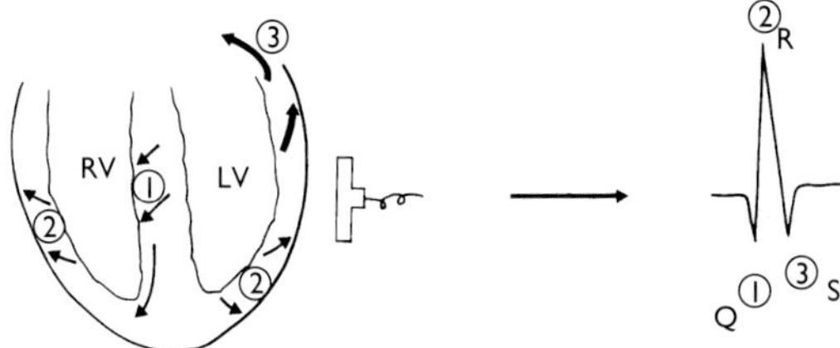

V_6 S wave after R wave as depolarisation spreads around ventricle away from V_6.

Left-ventricle hypertrophy (LVH)
V_5 or V_6—R wave >25 mm.
V_1 or V_2—S wave deep.
Tallest R wave + deepest S wave >35 mm.

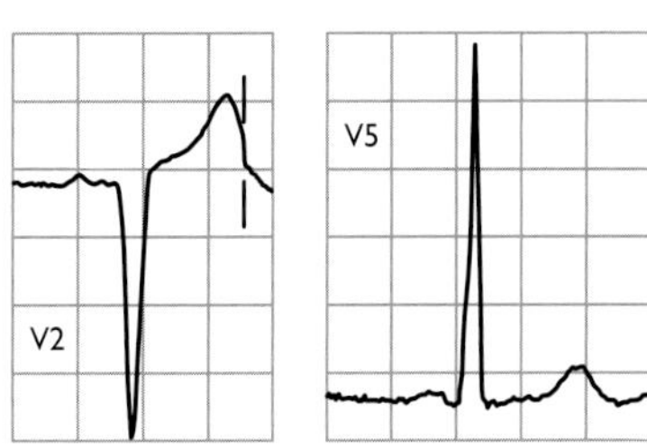

Left ventricular hypertrophy

- Voltage changes on their own are not enough—thin people with a thin ribcage can have big complexes.

- Obese people have small complexes.
- Also look for R wave in V_1—rotation to the right of transition point left axis deviation.
- T-wave inversion in V_5, V_6 in the presence of LVH is termed left ventricular 'strain pattern' and indicates marked hypertrophy.

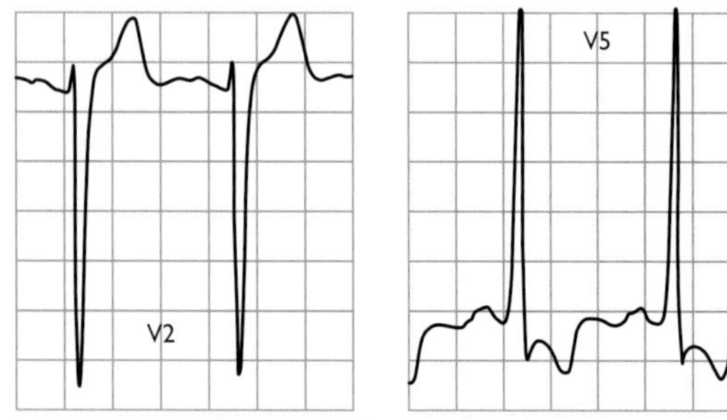

Left ventricular hypertrophy with strain

Right-ventricle hypertrophy (RVH)

The left ventricle is no longer dominant.

V_1—R wave > S wave.

V_6—deep S wave.

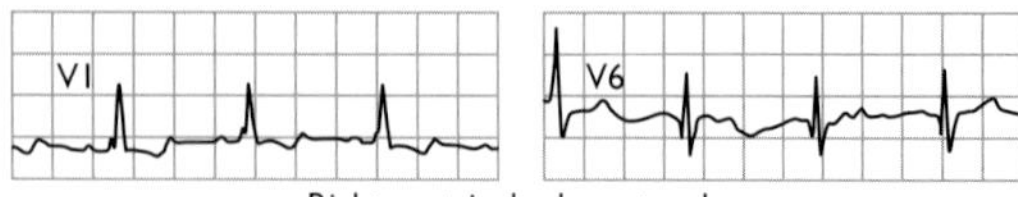

Right ventricular hypertrophy

- Also look for:
  - right axis deviation
  - peaked P of right atrial hypertrophy
  - T-wave inversion in V_2 and V_3—right ventricular 'strain pattern'.

Myocardial infarction (MI)—full thickness of ventricle

Infarction is the term for dead muscle.

Pathological Q wave:

- width = or >0.04 seconds (one small square)
- depth > one-third height of R wave

- smaller Q waves are physiological from septum depolarisation
- as ventricles depolarize from inside, an electrode in the ventricle cavity would record contraction as Q wave
- through 'dead' window, this is seen as if from inside the heart, i.e. the depolarisation of the far ventricle wall away from the electrode gives a negative deflection.

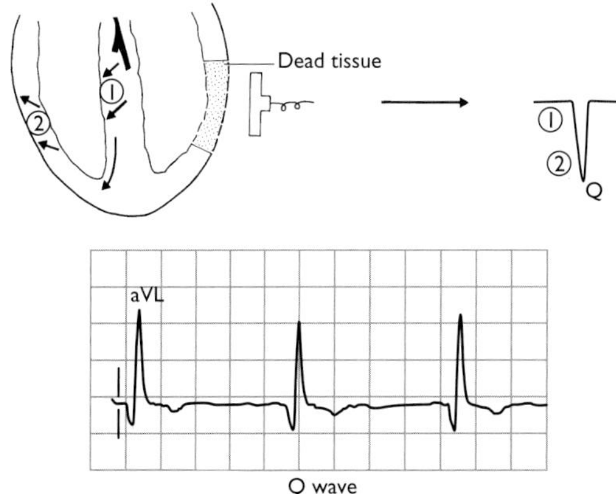

Acute myocardial ischaemia—raised ST segments

Damaged but potentially salvageable myocardium:

- ST segment—normally within 0.5 mm of isoelectric line
- ST elevation in V_1 and V_2 may be normal—high 'take-off' of j point
- ST elevation elsewhere is normal.

Normal baseline:

Resting myocardial cell potential approximately –90 mV. In an injured cell, failing cell membrane only allows potential of perhaps –40 mV.

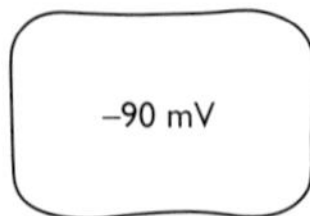

Resting potential in normal myocardial cell

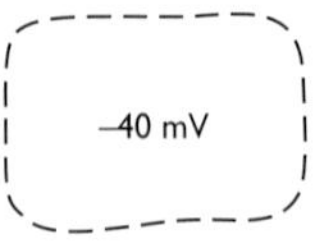

Resting potential in injured myocardial cell

If two electrodes record from different areas of the resting heart, one normal and one injured, a galvanometer would register –50 mV (i.e. the difference between –90 mV and –40 mV). This depresses the baseline below normal over the injured area, although this cannot be recognised until after QRS complex.

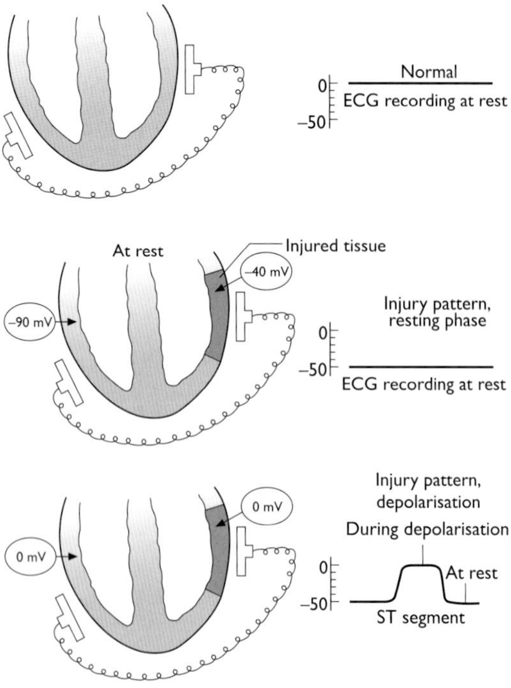

0
–50
Normal
ECG recording at rest

At rest
Injured tissue
–40 mV
–90 mV
Injury pattern, resting phase
0
–50
ECG recording at rest

0 mV
0 mV
Injury pattern, depolarisation
During depolarisation
0
–50
At rest
ST segment

Table 13.1 Classical time sequence of onset of ECG changes in myocardial infarction.

Approximate time of onset after chest pain	ECG changes
Immediately	ECG may be normal. Occasionally ST segment changes occur immediately pain develops, or even before
0–2 hours	ST segments rise—occluded artery → injury pattern
3–8 hours	Injured tissue remains Some dies (Q waves = myocardium death) Some improves to become ischaemic only (T-wave inversion) Full infarct pattern: • Q waves • raised ST segments • inverted T waves
8–24 hours	Injured tissue either dies → Q wave or improves and abnormal ST segments disappear Inverted T waves remain
After 1–2 days	Ischaemia disappears T waves upright again Q waves usually remain, as dead tissue will not not come alive again

Q waves may subsequently disappear if scarred tissue contracts.

Raised ST segment:

- acute ischaemic injury of ventricle
- pericarditis
- normal athletes
- normal West Indians.

Anterior infarction (Figures 13.2 and 13.3)

- changes in leads V_{1-6}
  - occlusion of left anterior descending coronary artery

Inferior infarction (Figure 13.4)

- changes in leads II, III, aVF
  - occlusion of right coronary artery

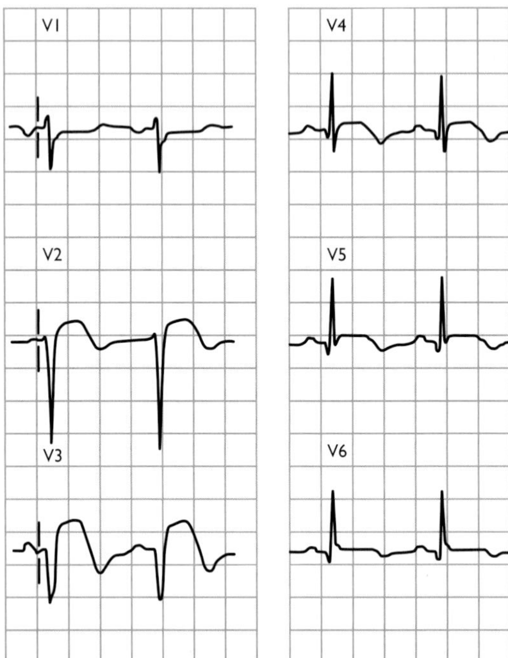

Figure 13.2 Acute anterior infarct: ST ↑ V_{2-6} at 3–8 hours.

Lateral infarction

- changes in leads I, aVL
  - occlusion of circumflex artery

Septal infarction

- changes in leads V_{2-3}
  - occlusion of septal branches of left anterior descending coronary artery

Posterior infarction

- changes in lead V_1 (e.g. R wave, ST depression)
  - occlusion of branches of right coronary artery

Chronic myocardial ischaemia

Reduced oxygen supply to muscle:

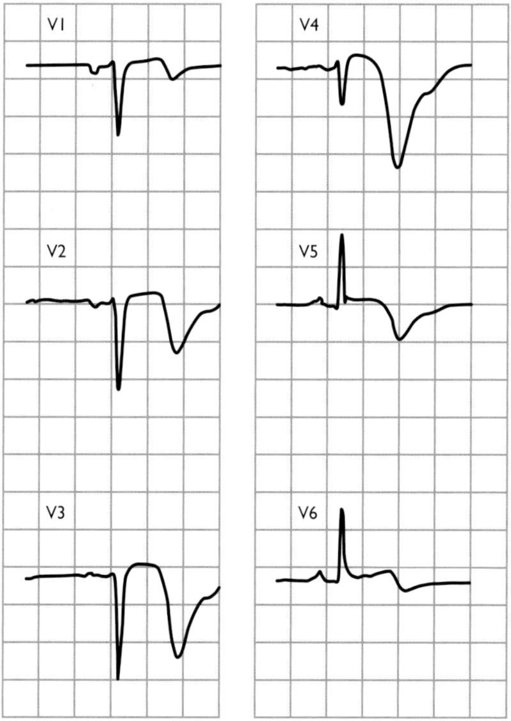

Figure 13.3 Ten hours after anterior myocardial infarct.

- ST depression
- T-wave inversion
- occasionally tall pointed T wave.

These changes can also occur during an exercise tolerance test when ischaemia develops:

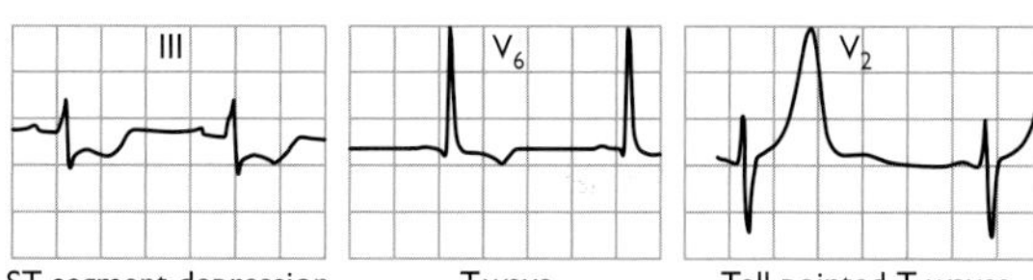

ST segment depression

T-wave inversion—ischaemic

Tall pointed T waves

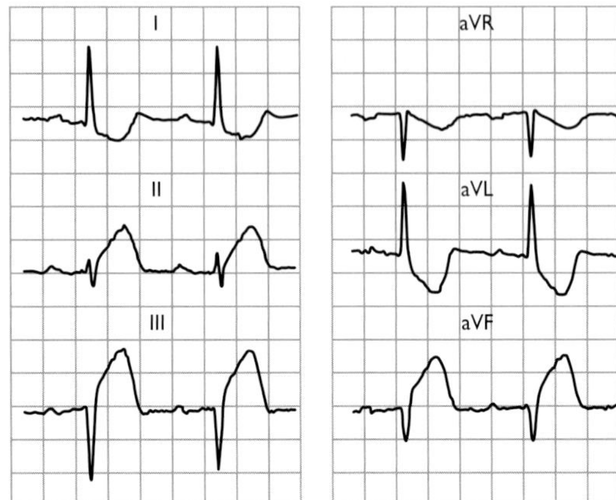

Figure 13.4 Acute inferior infarct: ST ↑ in II, III, a VF with reciprocal depression in other leads.

QRS axis

- The direction of depolarisation of the heart is sometimes helpful in diagnosis.
- Note the axis deviation on its own is rarely significant but alerts you to look for right or left ventricular hypertrophy.
- Look at the standard leads for the most equiphasic QRS complex (R and S equal). The axis is approximately at right angles to this in the direction of the most positive standard lead (largest R wave).

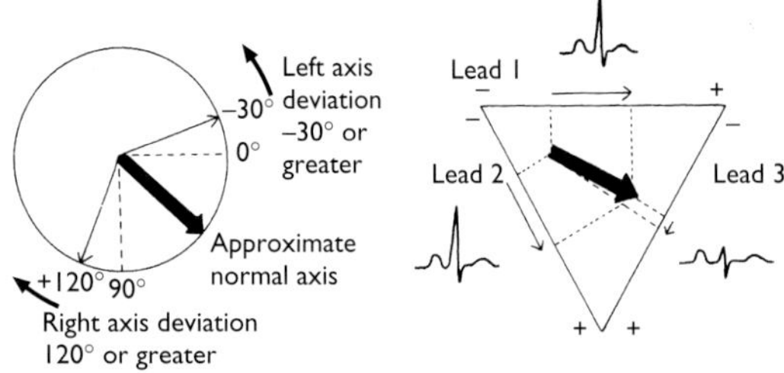

Pattern recognition

Left axis deviation

I /\ QRS complexes part like arms
III \/ of letter L

Lead II S = R implies –30°

Lead II S > R implies > –30°

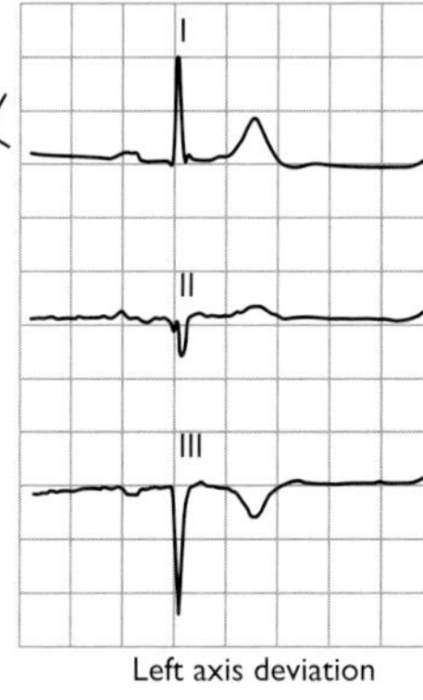

Left axis deviation

Right axis deviation

I \/ QRS complexes point together
III /\ like letter R

Lead I S = R implies +90°

Lead I S > R implies > +90°

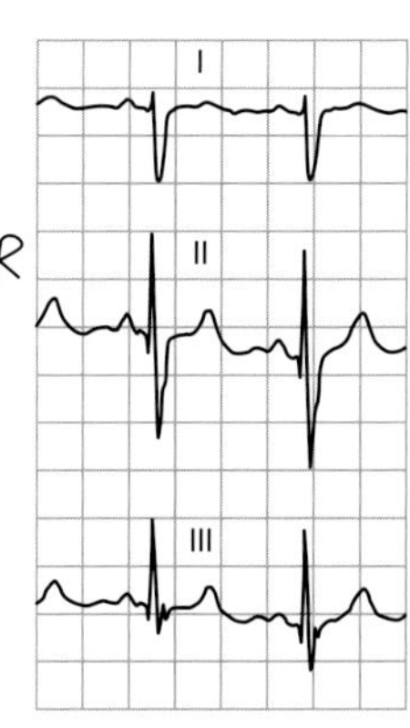

QRS complex

- Normal if width <0.12 second (three small squares).
- If >0.12 second—bundle-branch block.
- An apparently wide QRS complex, <0.12 second wide—partial bundle-branch block or interventricular conduction defect.
- Left bundle-branch block (LBBB) is usually associated with some form of heart disease.

- RBBB is often a normal variation, especially in athletes. Immediately after a myocardial infarction the development of RBBB may be serious.

Left bundle-branch block

- M pattern in V_6 (remember WiLLiaM).
- Throughout ECG, slurred ST segment and T wave inversion opposite to major deflection of QRS.
- Lead V_6
  - depolarisation of septal muscle from right bundle gives positive deflection
  - right heart depolarisation gives negative deflection
  - left heart depolarisation gives positive deflection.

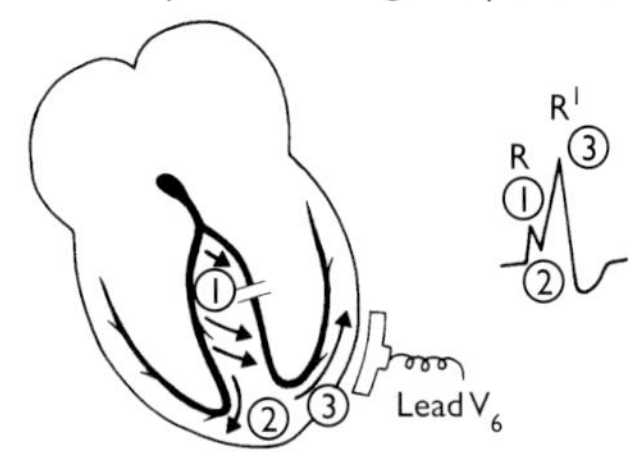

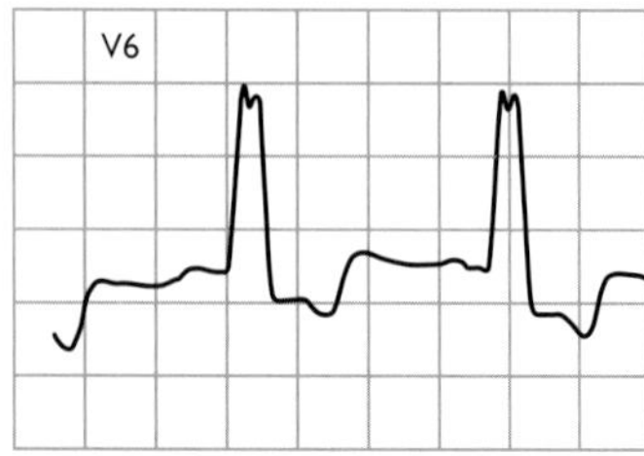

- Standard leads
  - left axis deviation as impulse spreads from right bundle up to left ventricle
  - also occurs if only anterior fascicle of left bundle blocked
  - left anterior hemiblock.

Right bundle-branch block

- M pattern in V_1 (remember MoRRoW).

* Lead V_1
    * depolarisation of septal muscle from left bundle gives positive deflection
    * left heart depolarisation gives negative deflection
    * right heart depolarisation gives positive deflection.

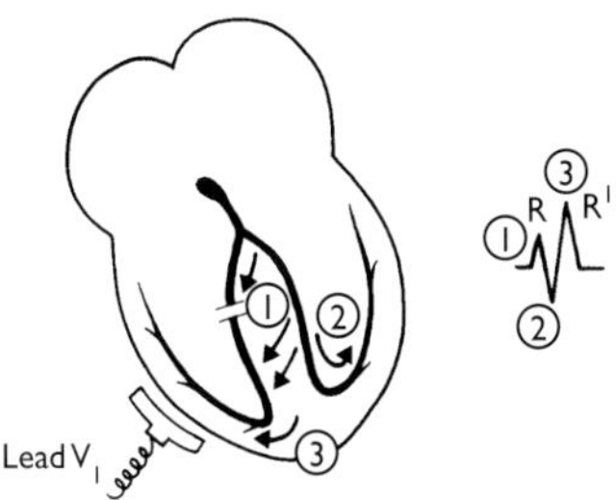

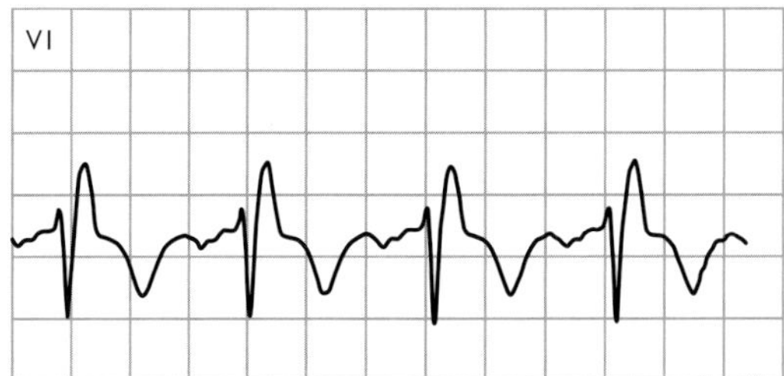

* Standard leads
    * axis usually normal, as depends on large muscle mass of left ventricle
    * if RBBB is associated with left axis, there is block of anterior fascicle of left bundle—bifascicular block

All heart is being excited via remaining posterior fascicle of left bundle.

Arrhythmias

* sinus arrhythmia
* ectopics
* tachycardias
* bradycardias

Sinus arrhythmia

Normal variation with respiratory rate—increase rate on inspiration.

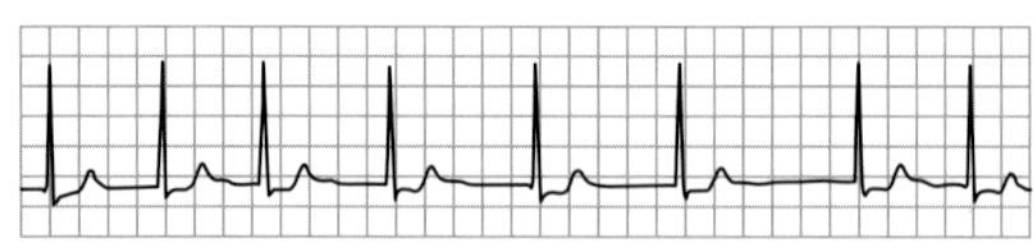

Ectopics

Atrial ectopics

Ectopic focus anywhere in atria. Depolarisation spreads across atrium to AV node like any normal beat:

- P wave is abnormal shape
- normal QRS complex.

The atrial ectopic focus must fire early—or would be entrained by normal excitation:

- appears early on rhythm strip
- followed by compensatory pause—waiting for normal SA node cycle.

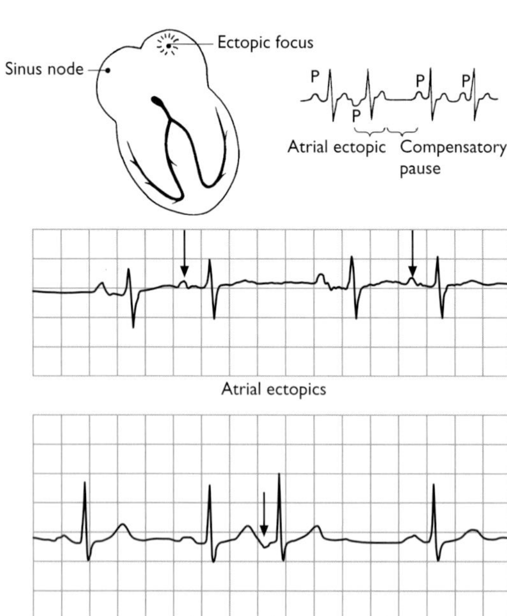

Atrial ectopics

Atrial ectopic—an inverted P wave

Junctional or nodal ectopics

Ectopic at AV node; no P wave.

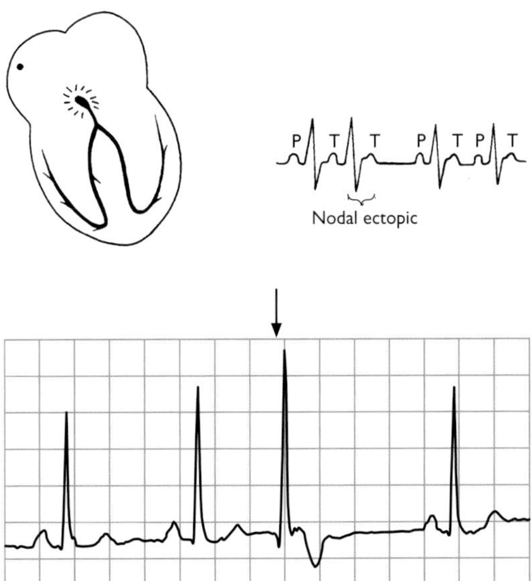

Ventricular ectopics

Ectopic anywhere in ventricles. Depolarisation occurs first in that ventricle then spreads to other ventricle:

- no P wave
- wide complex
- bundle branch-block pattern
  - left focus—RBBB pattern
  - right focus—LBBB pattern.

Atrial and junctional ectopics are invariably innocent when picked up on a random ECG. The majority of ventricular ectopics are also innocent except after a myocardial infarction. Ventricular ectopics picked up on routine monitoring of healthy patients are approximately proportional to age, i.e. 30% of 30-year-olds, 50% of 50-year-olds and almost 100% of 70-year-olds. Innocent ventricular ectopics usually disappear on exercise.

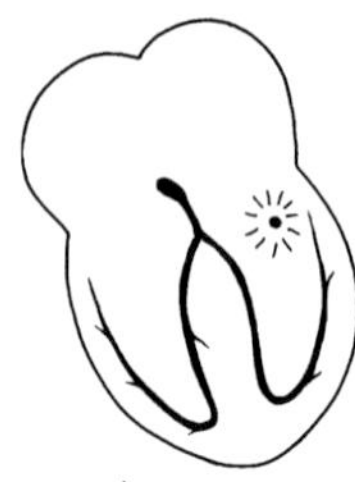

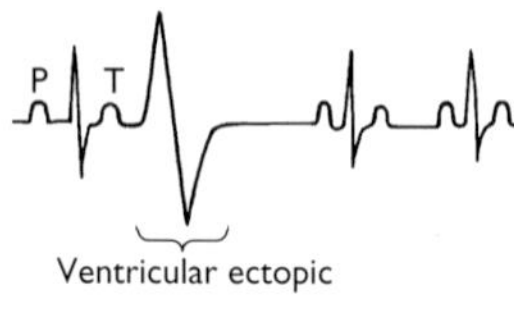

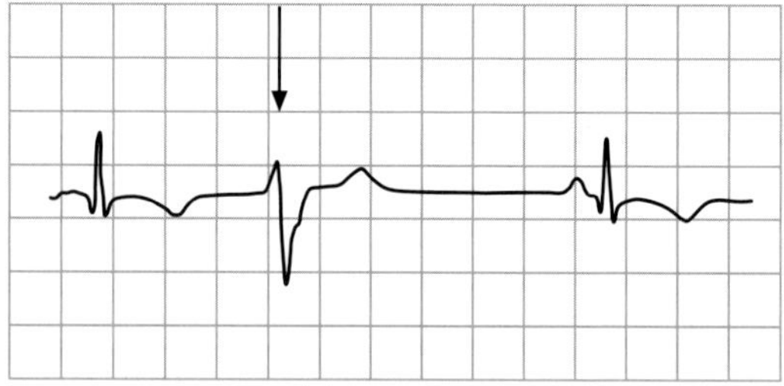

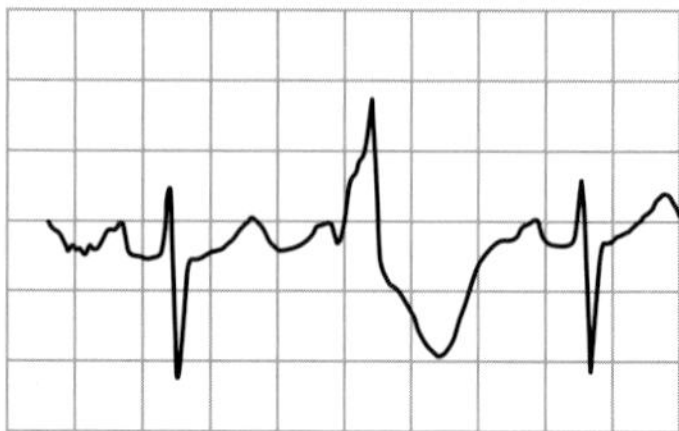

Tachycardias

Classification of tachycardias

- Tachycardias are divided into:
  - **Narrow-complex regular**—QRS complex up to 0.08 seconds—two little squares on ECG
    - sinus tachycardia
    - supraventricular tachycardia, atrial tachycardia, atrial flutter.

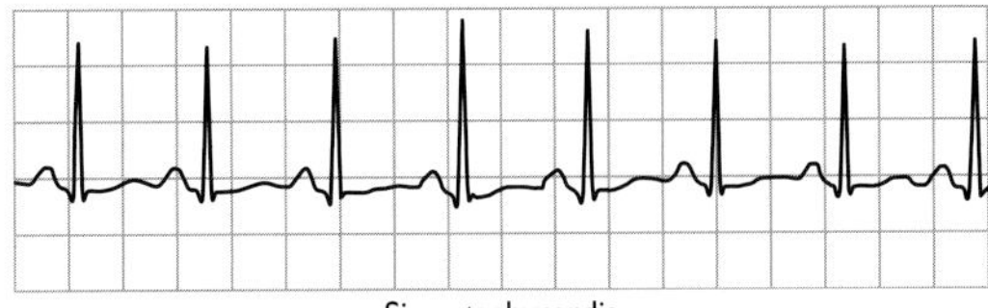
Sinus tachycardia

- **Narrow-complex irregular**
  - atrial tachycardia with varying block, atrial fibrillation.
- **Broad-complex**—QRS complex about 0.12 seconds—three small squares
  - ventricular arrhythmias and occasionally supraventricular with aberrant (delayed) conduction.

- Deciding whether a tachycardia is **atrial** or **ventricular** is not easy. Here are some pointers.
  - Narrow-complex tachycardias are usually atrial and broad-complex usually ventricular, **but not always**.
  - When acute ischaemic heart disease is present, tachycardias are usually ventricular. In the absence of ischaemic heart disease tachycardias are usually atrial, **but not always**.
  - If there is independent atrial activity (random appearance of p values), the tachycardia is ventricular.
  - Look at the patient's preceding ECGs or rhythm strip. If the tachycardia looks like a previous ectopic beat in shape, it will be that type of tachycardia.
  - Vagal stimulation (rubbing carotid, etc.) will only be effective in atrial rhythms.
  - The regularity or irregularity is not helpful in distinguishing ventricular from atrial arrhythmias.

Atrial fibrillation

The electrical impulse and contraction travel randomly around the atria:

- 'bag-of-worms' quivering atria
- irregular little waves on ECG—best seen V_1.

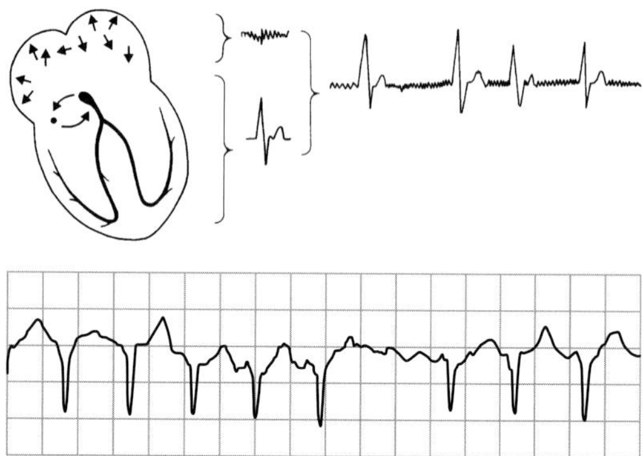

When it first develops, often 150+, fibrillation waves are difficult to see:

- AV node fires irregularly
- normal QRS complexes.

If irregular rate, no P waves, normal QRS—likely to be atrial fibrillation.

Digoxin is still the drug of choice—it decreases transmission of impulses down the bundle of His.

Atrial flutter

Atria contract very rapidly, 200–250 beats/min, giving a sawtooth pattern, but the ventricles only respond to every second or third or fourth contraction (2 : 1, 3 : 1, 4 : 1 block).

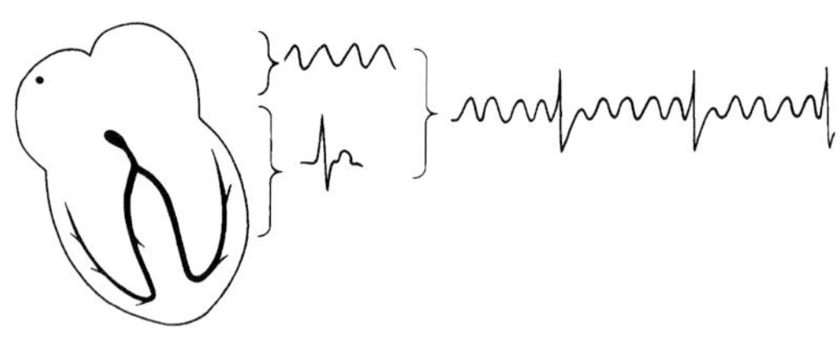

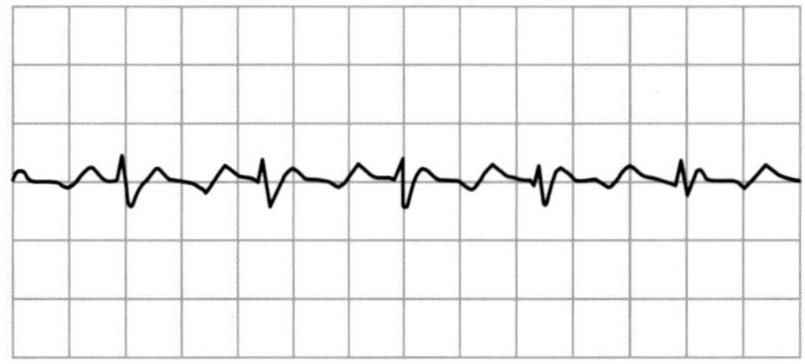

2 : 1 atrial flutter

Treated with digoxin, normally changes to atrial fibrillation.

Supraventricular tachycardia (SVT)

- Arises near AV node, 170 beats/min or more, regular.
- Complexes are identical, normal width or wide if also bundle-branch block.
- Common in young patients (20–30 years).
- Rarely represents heart disease.
- Sudden onset and finish.
- Lasts few minutes to several hours.
- May be tired, light-headed, uncomfortable.
- In older patients SVTs more likely to represent heart disease.

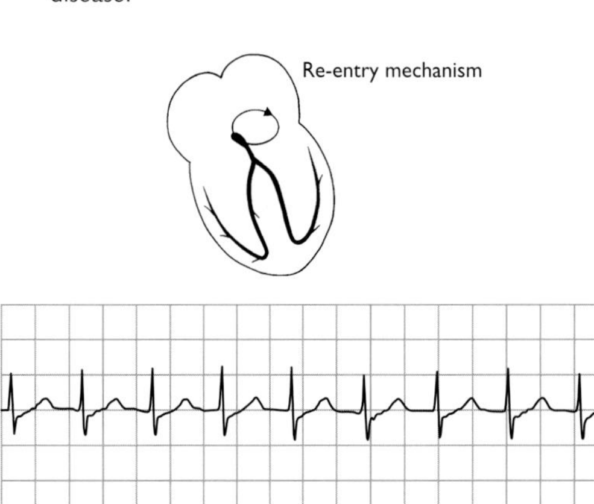

Vagal stimulation (rubbing carotid sinus) can terminate attack.

Re-entry is the most common mechanism for tachycardias (Figure 13.5). Assumes two conduction pathways lead to ventricles. Normally conduction passes equally quickly down both pathways.

Problems arise when one pathway recovers more slowly than the other. When this happens the next conduction passes down only one pathway.

Conduction subsequently passes retrogradely up the other pathway, which is no longer refractory. This pathway then becomes refractory while the first pathway conducts again and the impulse races round the pathways to give a tachycardia.

Wolff–Parkinson–White syndrome

This is the classic re-entry arrhythmia. There are two separate pathways from the atria to the ventricles. In

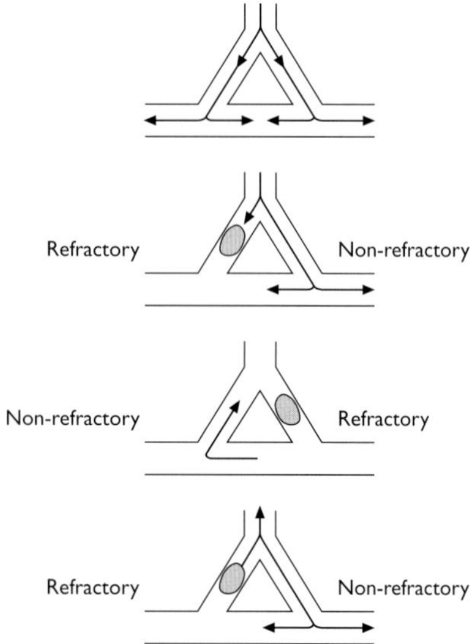

Figure 13.5 The mechanism of re-entry tachycardias.

the resting ECG the early entry, by the aberrant conduction pathway bypassing the bundle of His, is seen as a delta wave.

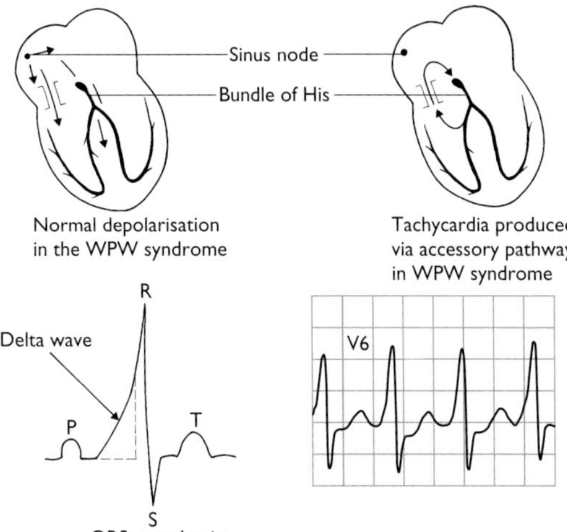

Ventricular tachycardia

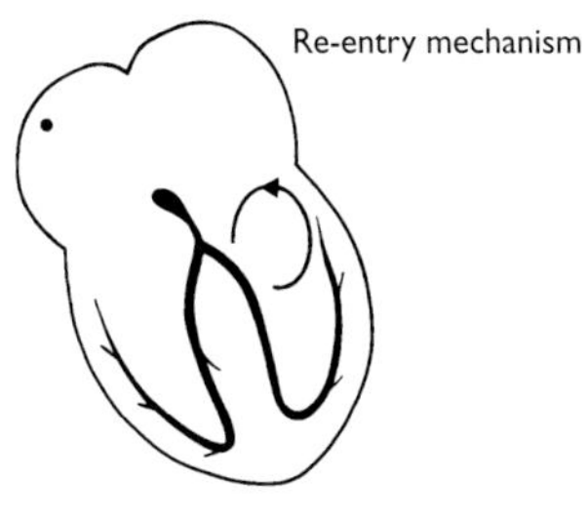

- Potentially dangerous rhythm which can develop into ventricular fibrillation.
- Rapid but not as fast as SVT (usually less than 170 beats/min).
- Often slightly irregular.
- Patient often looks collapsed.

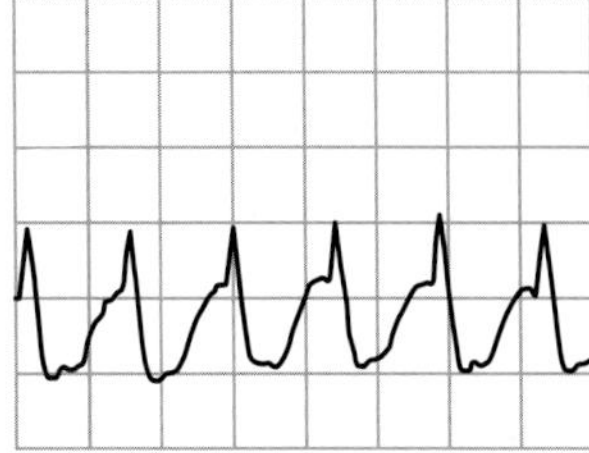

- Always wide QRS complex:
  - LBBB pattern—right focus
  - RBBB pattern—left focus.

Treatment is with amiodarone intravenously, DC cardioversion or overdrive pacing at once with transfer of the patient to hospital.

Bradycardias

Pulse rate <60 beats/min.

Sinus

Normal P wave and QRS complexes.

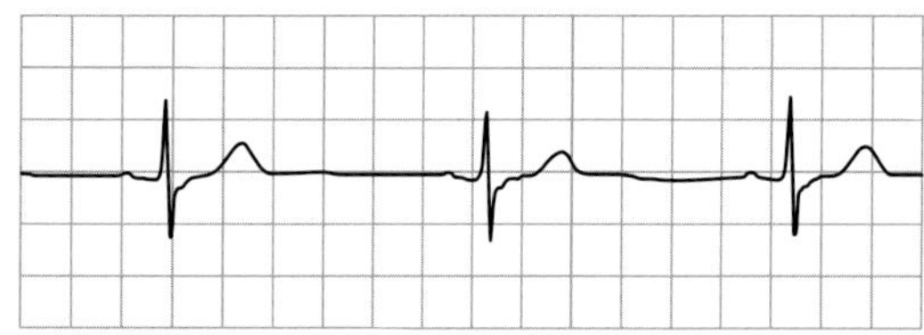

Sinus bradycardia

- **Causes:**
  - athletic heart
  - β-blockers
  - hypothyroidism
  - raised intracranial pressure
  - pain with vagal response
    - dental pain
    - glaucoma
    - biliary colic.

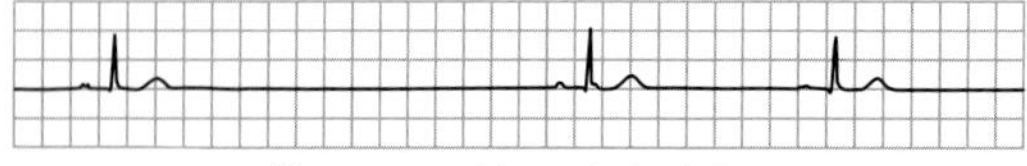

Sinus arrest with vagal stimulation

First-degree heart block

- PR interval (beginning of P wave to beginning of QRS complex) >0.22 second (5.5 little squares).
- Depolarization delayed in the region of AV node.

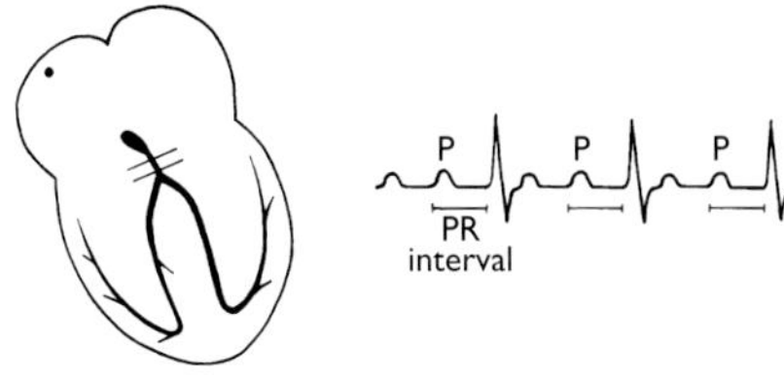

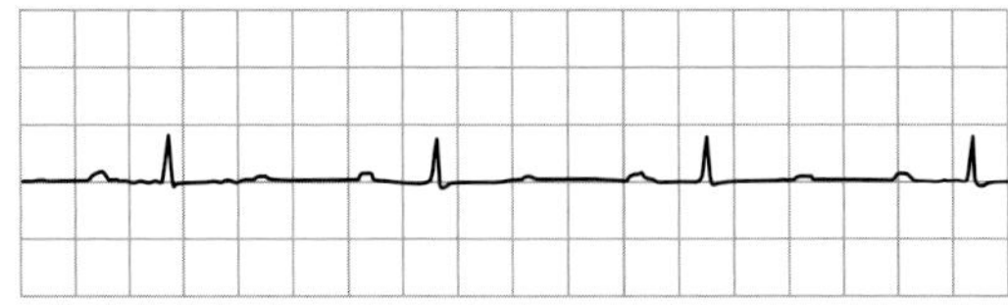

Wenckebach heart block
In a cycle of three or four beats the PR interval gradually lengthens until a P wave appears on its own with no QRS complex. The cycle then repeats itself.

P P P P P P
PR
interval

Gradually increasing PR interval until a QRS is dropped

2:1 Block
The QRS complexes only respond to every other P wave, i.e. every other P wave has no QRS complex.

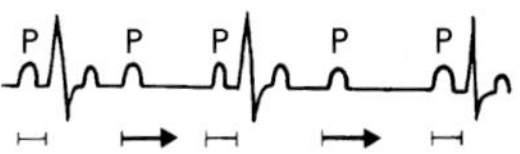

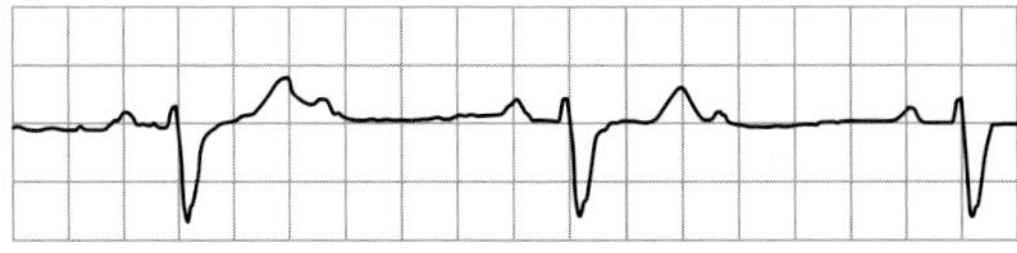

2 : 1 heart block

Complete heart block

- No relation between P waves and QRS complex.
- Inherent ventricular rate about 40 beats/min.
- QRS complex abnormal as it arises in a ventricular focus.

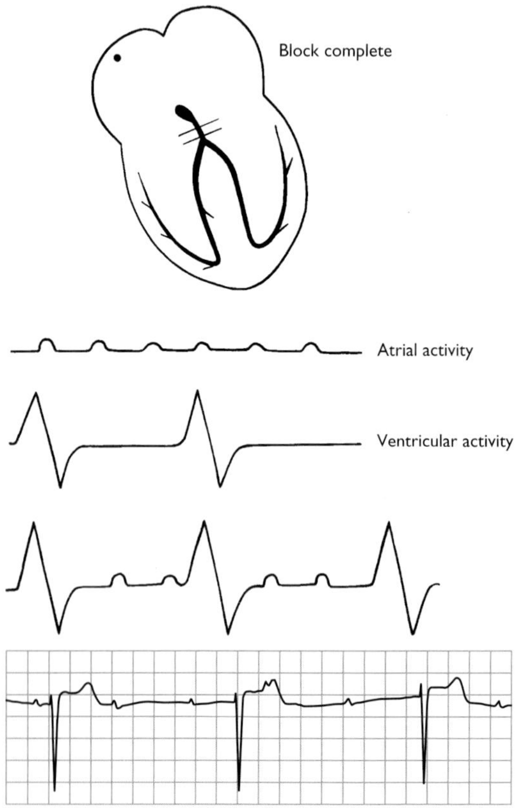

Complete heart block

Pacemakers

- When conduction defects cause asystolic pauses or very slow heart rates, pacemakers can

stimulate either the atrium or ventricle and restore rhythm.
- Pacemakers can be basic or very sophisticated.

Ventricle-only pacemakers

These are the commonest types of pacemaker (80%+). If the ventricle fails to produce an electrical signal (QRS complex), the pacemaker senses this and fires at approximately 60–70 beats/min. It is inhibited when the ventricles QRS complex returns at an adequate rate.

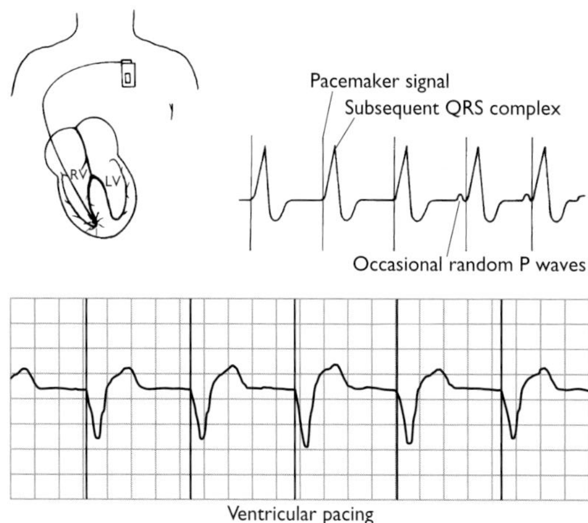

Ventricular pacing

Atrial-only pacemakers

In the sick sinus syndrome, the P wave fails to materialise but conduction in the AV node and bundle of His is normal. Pacing the atrium restores normal function.

Sequential pacemakers

These pacemakers cause the sequential contraction of the atrium and ventricle in a more normal physiological way. This may provide a better cardiac output.

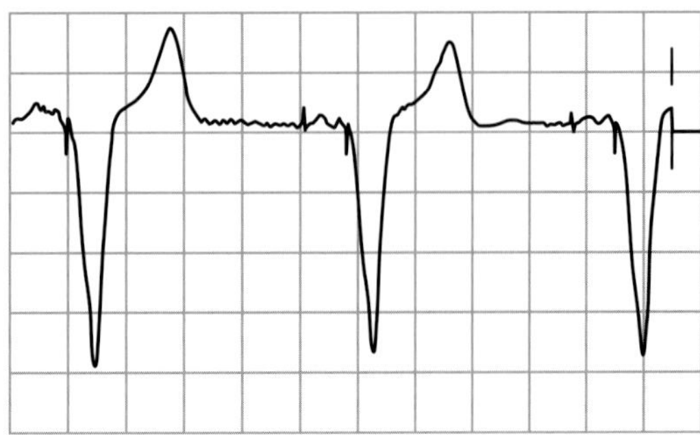

Sequential pacing

Looking at the ECG

Examine logically, reading complexes from left to right. Remember to identify the patient correctly and check the date and time. Often there may be a note on the ECG to say whether the patient was in pain at the time or not.

- **Rhythm:**
  - sinus rhythm ± ectopics. Ignore sinus arrhythmia
  - regular
    - slow complete heart block
    - sinus bradycardia
    - fast sinus tachycardia
    - supraventricular tachycardia
    - ventricular tachycardia
    - regular atrial flutter
  - irregular
    - atrial fibrillation
    - atrial tachycardia with varying block.
- **Rate:** add up the number of large squares between two successive beats. Divide into 300. For example:

$$\frac{300}{5 \text{ large squares}} = 60 \text{ beats/min}$$

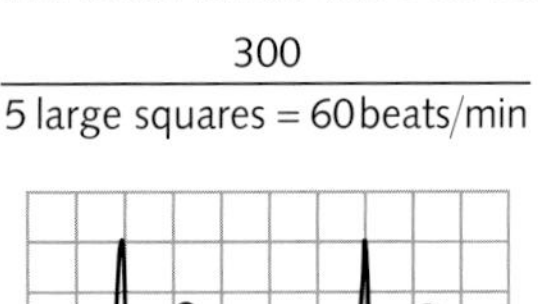

1.5 squares	= 200 beats/min	3.5	= 85 beats/min
2	= 150 beats/min	4	= 75 beats/min
2.5	= 120 beats/min	5	= 60 beats/min
3	= 100 beats/min	6	= 50 beats/min

If the simple formula does not work for irregular rhythm—then add up number of complexes in 6 seconds (sometimes marked on the paper) and multiply by 10.

- **Complex shape**—brief guide:
  - P wave: abnormal shape
    - atrial ectopics, P mitrale, P pulmonale
    - 0.10–0.22 second (2.5–5.5 squares)
  - PR interval: prolonged
    - >0.22 second: first-degree heart block
    - <0.1 second: Wolff–Parkinson–White syndrome
  - QRS complex
    - large Q wave—full-thickness infarct?
    - wide QRS >0.12 second: branch block
    - R wave if large: ventricular hypertrophy?
  - ST segment: elevated or depressed—ischaemia or other causes?
  - T wave: if inverted—ischaemia or other causes?

In summary, particularly look for:
- abnormal rhythm
- abnormal rate
- abnormal QRS—especially ischaemia, infarct, hypertrophy.

Exercise electrocardiography (stress testing)

- Exercise may reveal cardiac dysfunction not apparent at rest.
- Most commonly used in suspected coronary artery disease.

Connected to a 12-lead electrocardiograph (ECG) machine, with resuscitation equipment available, the patient exercises at an increasing workload on a treadmill (or bicycle). **Bruce protocol**: 3-minute stages of increasing belt speed and treadmill gradient. Take ECG every minute, blood pressure every 3 minutes.

This assesses:

- exercise capacity
- haemodynamic response
- symptoms
- ECG changes.

Exercise for as long as possible stopping when there are:

- marked symptoms
- severe ECG changes
- ventricular arrhythmias
- fall in blood pressure.

Myocardial ischaemia causes ST segment depression. A high false-positive rate occurs in absence of angina (about 20%). False-positive incidence depends on age and sex, with young females having the highest rate, even in the presence of typical symptoms of angina.

Clinically important abnormalities are:

- horizontal or downward sloping ST depression (Figure 13.6)
- deep ST depression
- ST changes with typical anginal symptoms.

A definitely negative test at a high workload denotes an excellent prognosis.

- **Angiography is indicated** if only a low workload is achieved before important abnormalities occur.
- **Medical treatment of angina** may be appropriate if three or four stages are completed.

Echocardiography

This visualises structures and function of the heart. It uses ultrasound (2.5–7.5 MHz) to reflect from interfaces in the heart, e.g. ventricle and atrial walls, heart, valves, major vessels. The higher frequency gives better discrimination but lower tissue penetration. The time delay between transmission and reception indicates depth. The usual approach is transthoracic (TEE), but transoesophageal

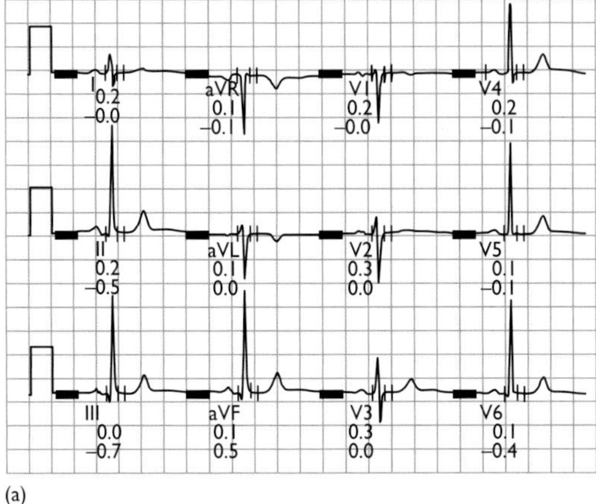

(a)

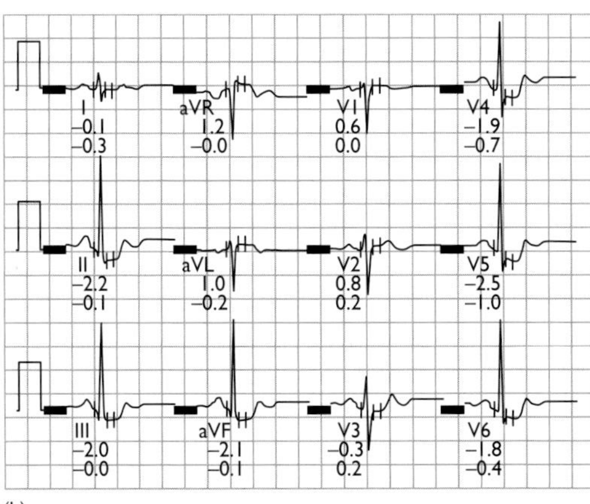

(b)

Figure 13.6 Example of a strongly positive exercise test—signal averaged recordings before exercise (a) and at peak effort (b). There is a marked horizontal ST depression in the inferolateral leads, II, III, aVF and V4–6.

echocardiography (TOE), involving sedation of the patient and insertion of an endoscope probe into the oesophagus, gives more detailed views.

Two-dimensional echocardiography

2D echocardiography (Figure 13.7) uses a scanning beam swept backwards and forwards across a 45° or 60° arc to construct a picture of the anatomy of the heart.

2D echocardiography is excellent for demonstrating:

- valvular anatomy
- ventricular function, e.g. poor contraction, low ejection fraction, akinetic segment, paradoxical motion in aneurysm

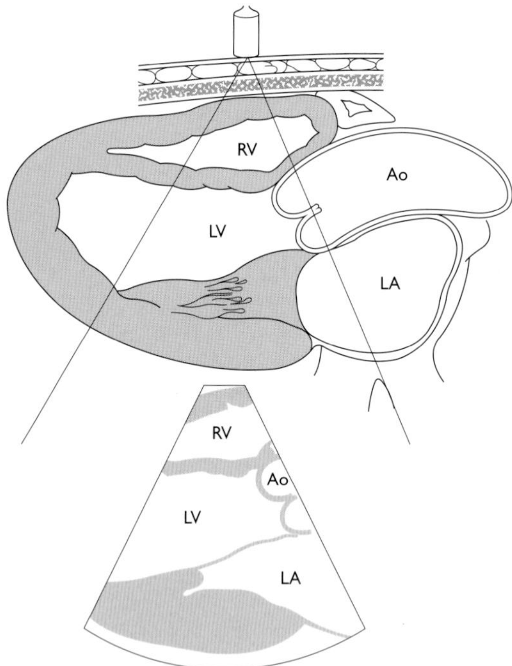

Figure 13.7 Two-dimensional echocardiograph. Ao = aorta; LA = left atrium; LV = left ventricle; RV = right ventricle.

- structural abnormalities:
  - pericardial effusion
  - ventricular hypertrophy
  - congenital heart disease.

Quantifying valvular function is better achieved by Doppler echocardiography.

M-mode echocardiography

M-mode echocardiography (Figure 13.8) uses a single pencil beam, and movements of the heart in that beam are visualised on moving sensitised paper. It predates 2D echocardiography but is useful for measuring ventricular diameters in systole/diastole.

Radionuclide imaging in cardiology

Radionuclides can be used in the assessment of cardiac disease in three main ways.

Myocardial perfusion scintigraphy

- **Demonstrates abnormal blood flow in coronary artery disease** in conjunction with exercise testing.

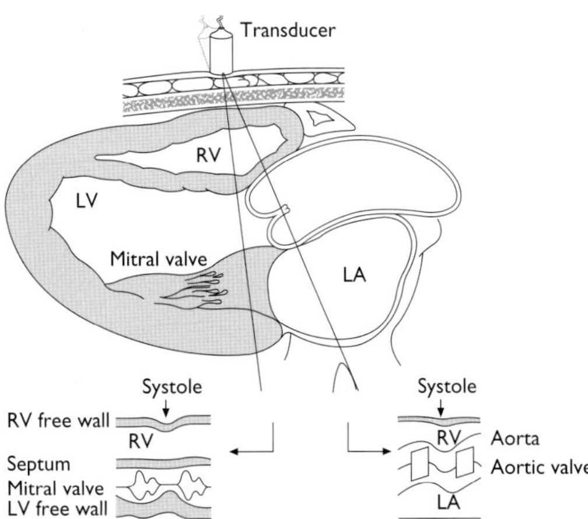

Figure 13.8 M-mode echocardiographs, with two examples showing mitral and aortic valves opening and closing. LA = left atrium; LV = left ventricle; RV = right ventricle.

Thallium 201 is extracted from the blood in proportion to flow.

- Ischaemic myocardium appears as a cold spot on the scan taken immediately after injection of thallium.
- If the area is not infarcted, the cold spot 'fills in' as thallium redistributes in the following 4 hours.
- Thallium scanning is a more reliable diagnostic investigation than exercise testing and the number and extent of defects correlate with prognosis.

Radionuclide ventriculography (multiple gated acquisition (MUGA) scanning)

- Assesses ventricle function.

The patient's blood (usually red blood cells) is labelled with technetium 99 m (half-life 6 hours). A gamma camera and a computer generate a moving image of the heart by 'gating' the computer to the patient's ECG.

Systolic function of the left ventricle is quantified by the ejection fraction (normally 0.50–0.70):

$$\text{Ejection fraction} = \frac{\text{stroke volume}}{\text{end-diastolic volume}},$$

i.e. the proportion of the total diastolic volume that is ejected in systole.

Images can be collected during exercise as well as at rest, to assess the effect of stress on left ventricular function.

Pyrophosphate scanning

- Demonstrates recent myocardial infarction, e.g. 1–10 days after event.

Technetium 99 m pyrophosphate is taken up by areas of myocardial infarction producing a hot spot, maximal at 3 days.

Indicated when:

- the ECG is too abnormal to demonstrate infarction (e.g. left bundle-branch block)
- the patient has presented after the plasma enzyme changes, e.g. at 3 days.

Doppler ultrasound cardiography

- Velocity of blood movement in the heart and circulation assessed by Doppler shift.
- Blood accelerates through an obstruction, e.g. a stenosed valve. The peak velocity is proportional to the haemodynamic gradient.
- Reverse flow pattern in valvular reflux.

Multigated Doppler or colour-flow Doppler

- Rapid method of detecting abnormal blood flow due to a leaking valve or an intracardiac shunt, e.g. ventricular septal defect.

Doppler ultrasound provides functional assessment to complement the anatomical assessment of 2D echocardiography.

- Echo machine calculates the direction and velocity of flow, pixel by pixel, within a segment of the image and codes it in colour.
- It superimposes flow on the 2D image.

Cardiac catheterisation

An invasive assessment of cardiac function and disease in which fine tubes are passed, with mild sedation under operating theatre conditions:

- retrograde through arteries to left side of heart and coronary arteries
- anterograde through veins to right side of heart and pulmonary arteries
  - to make diagnosis, e.g. is valve critically stenosed?
  - is chest pain due to coronary artery disease?
  - to plan cardiac surgery, particularly coronary artery bypass grafting.

It entails a major radiation dose.

Major complications (one in 2000 cases) include:

- access artery dissection (2%)
- myocardial infarction (0.1%)

- air or cholesterol emboli, which can cause stroke or myocardial infarction
- death (0.01%).

Risks must be outweighed by the benefit the patient receives.

The commonest approach is **cannulation of the right femoral vessels by the Seldinger technique**. A percutaneous fine gauge needle punctures the vessel, through which a soft guide wire is passed. The needle is withdrawn and an introducer sheath and catheter is inserted over the guide wire, which is then withdrawn. Haemostasis is achieved by compression. The technique is not suitable if the patient is on anticoagulant drugs, has severe peripheral vascular disease or an abdominal aortic aneurysm.

Alternative approach: **brachial vessels at elbow through a skin incision**. Closure of arterotomy by sutures allows use in anticoagulated patients.

If stenosis is found in the coronary arteries then it may be amenable to percutaneous transluminal coronary angioplasty (PTCA) either with balloon or stent.

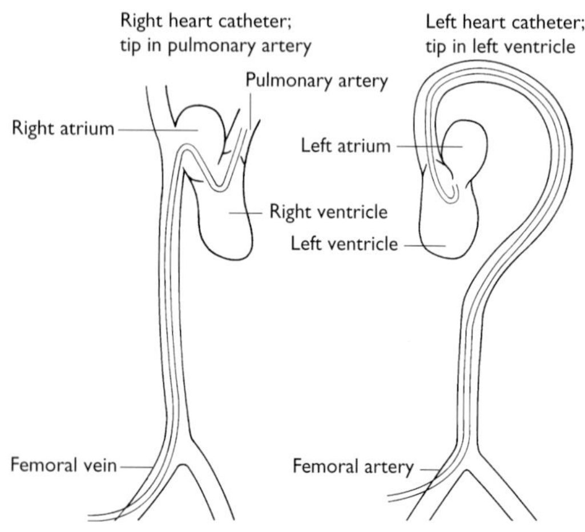

Pressure measurements

Cardiac haemodynamics and gradients across individual valves, e.g. by pulling the catheter back across the **aortic valve**, while systolic pressure is recorded (Figure 13.9).

Mitral stenosis is quantified by the diastolic pressure difference between the left ventricle (**left heart catheter**) and left atrium measured indirectly via the **right heart catheter** in the 'wedge' position—passed through the pulmonary artery to occlude a pulmonary arteriole so the pressure at the tip reflects the left atrial pressure transmitted through the pulmonary capillaries (Figure 13.10).

The **cardiac output** is calculated either by the **Fick principle** (cardiac output is inversely proportional to difference between systemic arterial and mixed venous blood oxygen saturation) or by the **thermodilution** technique.

Radio-opaque contrast

Radio-opaque contrast (iodine-based) is:

- injected into chambers to assess their systolic function and to detect valve regurgitation, e.g. left ventricular injection for mitral regurgitation
- injected into coronary ostia with multiple X-ray picture projections to detect coronary artery disease.

24-hour ECG tape recording

ECG worn for 24 hours (or 48 hours) (Figure 13.11); obtains on tape a continuous ECG recording during normal activities. For less frequent events longer periods may be recorded using subcutaneously implanted or clip-on recorders to record heart tracings.

For diagnosis of:

- palpitations
- dizzy spells
- light-headedness or black-outs of possible cardiac origin.

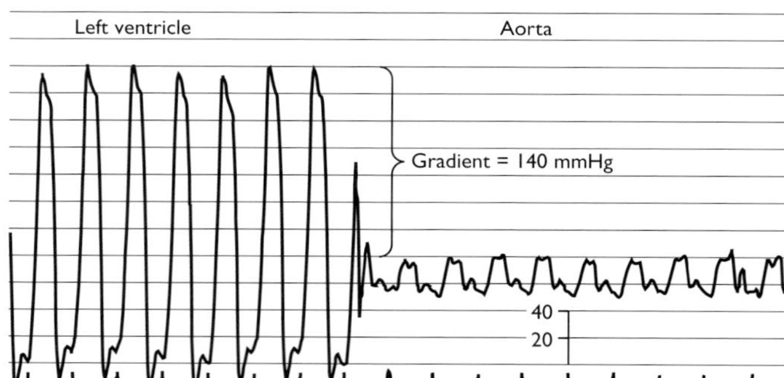

Figure 13.9 Aortic stenosis. The systolic pressure falls as the catheter tip leaves the left ventricle, crossing the stenosed aortic valve. Diastolic pressure is prevented from falling by the aortic valve.

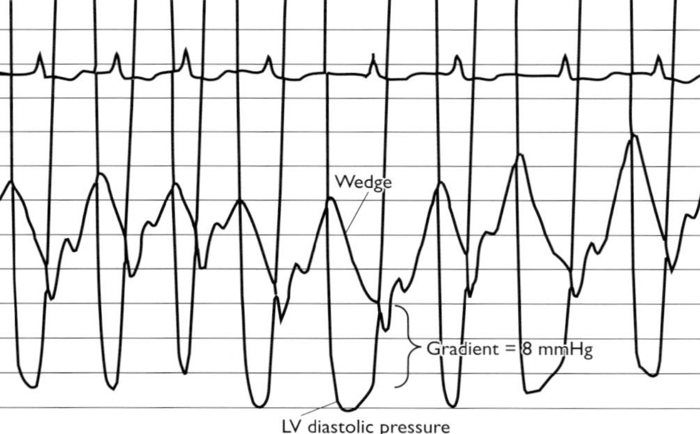

Figure 13.10 Mitral stenosis. Left ventricular (LV) pressure trace expanded to show low diastolic pressures. A pressure difference between the wedge trace and LV diastolic trace reflects obstruction to flow into the left ventricle due to mitral stenosis. The rhythm is atrial fibrillation.

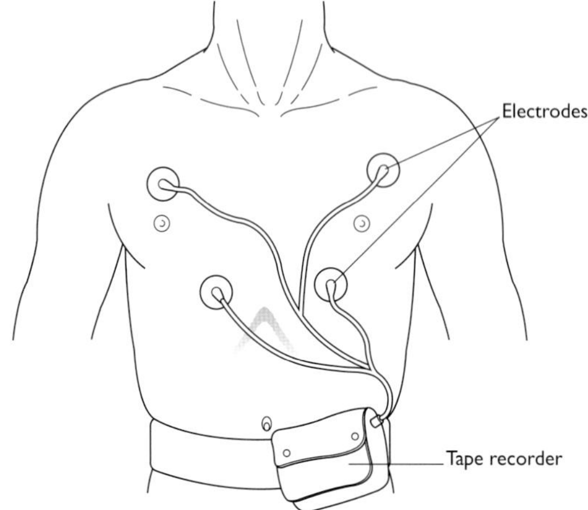

Figure 13.11 Arrangement for the 24-hour ECG tape recorder.

May show episodes of:

- atrial asystole
- atrial or ventricular tachycardias
- complete heart block
- ST segment changes during angina or silent ischaemia

However, often the most important finding is of no relation between ECG abnormalities and events.

24-hour blood pressure recording

Blood pressure is measured intermittently with an upper arm cuff and microphone, with recording on a tape. Allows evaluation of blood pressure during everyday activities without the 'white coat' effect of anxiety at the doctor's surgery increasing measured blood pressure. Hypertension is defined as daytime average >140/>90 mmHg. Absence of lower blood pressure during the night ('dip') suggests secondary hypertension.

CHAPTER 14
Practical skills

Measurement of blood pressure
Learning objectives
1 To be able to measure arterial blood pressure reliably and reproducibly in a normal patient using a mercury sphygmomanometer.
2 To describe the potential sources of artefact and how to avoid them.
3 To record findings in the patient's charts or notes.

Arterial blood pressure is traditionally measured at the brachial artery. Although aneroid and electronic devices are increasingly used, they are unreliable in the context of hypotension and dysrhythmias and it is essential that you are able to palpate the peripheral pulses and measure blood pressure manually with a mercury sphygmomanometer.
- Explain to the patient what you are about to do and why.
- Be aware of 'white coat hypertension' and allow the patient to sit or lie comfortably for a period before measurement.
- Expose and position the patient's arm palm upwards and wrap the cuff snugly around the arm, 2 cm above the antecubital fossa. The cuff should be large enough to allow the Velcro portions to be correctly opposed. A cuff that bulges and slips on inflation is either too small or inadequately applied, or both.

Clinical Skills and Examination: The Core Curriculum. By R Turner, B Angus, A Handa, C Hatton. ©2009 Blackwell Publishing, ISBN: 9781405157513.

- The sphygmomanometer is positioned at (your) eye level to avoid parallax. Contrary to popular dogma, it does not need to be level with the patient's heart.
- Inflate cuff until the radial pulse can no longer be felt. This provides an estimation of systolic pressure. Deflate the cuff completely and wait 15 to 30 seconds before continuing to measure.
- Palpate the brachial pulse. The cuff is then inflated to a pressure 30 mmHg higher than the estimated systolic pressure. Place the bell of the stethoscope over the brachial artery. Deflate the cuff at 5 mmHg per second. Record the systolic and diastolic pressures, along with the date, and compare the present reading with the previous readings.
- If clinically indicated, repeat on other arm.
- Remove the equipment and clean after use.

Measurement of pulse rate and characteristics

Learning objectives

1. To be able to locate and palpate the radial, brachial, carotid, femoral and pedal pulses.
2. To be able to describe the rate and character of the peripheral pulse.
3. To be able to infer the presence of disease states from your findings.

The radial pulse is the most readily accessible and serves as a window on the circulation in the majority of cases. It is palpated with the fingers, as is the femoral. The carotid and brachial pulses are palpated with the thumb. These major arteries are used to assess the circulation in shocked or collapsed patients.

- **Pulse rate**. For the student it is good practice to measure the pulse rate over a period of at least 15 seconds and to record the rate precisely. Tachycardia and bradycardia are generally defined as rates >100 and <50 min^{-1} respectively. If you use these descriptive terms, it implies that you are inferring something from your findings, and so you should be prepared to substantiate them.

- **Pulse rhythm**.
  - *Sinus arrhythmia*—acceleration in inspiration and deceleration in expiration—is the commonest cause of variance. It is normal and occurs in young fit people. The phenomenon is lost in heart failure and autonomic neuropathy.
  - *Ectopic beats* occur prematurely and so the pulse volume is smaller. The following normal beat occurs after a compensatory pause and so is of a fuller volume. These may be indicative of ischaemic heart disease.
  - *Atrial fibrillation* is characterised by an irregularly irregular pulse. With a rapid rate, some pulses may be too weak to palpate, and the true ventricular rate is determined by auscultation. The difference between this rate, and that counted at the wrist is the 'pulse deficit'.
- **Pulse volume and character** (determined from brachial or carotid).
  - *Pulse volume* reflects stroke volume. It is diminished in tachycardia and with poor ventricular function.
  - *Pulsus paradoxus* is an exaggerated fall in systolic pressure and pulse volume on inspiration. It occurs in severe asthma and with cardiac effusion and tamponade.
  - *Delayed pulse* occurs with obstruction to blood flow between the heart and periphery. In coarctation of the aorta the femoral pulses are delayed relative to the radial pulses.
  - *Slow rising pulse* occurs in aortic stenosis and so may be accompanied by a palpable thrill.
  - *Collapsing pulse* is characterised by a full and rapid rise followed by a rapid fall, and occurs in aortic regurgitation. This is accentuated by raising the patient's arm (after checking the manoeuvre will not cause pain).

Measurement of jugular venous pressure

Learning objectives

1 To understand and be able to describe the utility of measuring JVP.
2 To be able to measure JVP reliably and reproducibly.
3 To be able to infer the presence of disease states from your findings.

JVP and CVP are estimates of right atrial filling pressure and serve as a proxy for left atrial filling pressure. They indicate ventricular preload and are useful in examining the adequacy of ventricular function and in titrating fluid or diuretic therapy in either 'shocked' or 'fluid overloaded' patients. A JVP of 7 cm corresponds to a CVP of about 5 mmHg, which is normal.

- Explain to the patient what you are about to do and why.
- Sit the patient reclining at 45°.
- Identify the *internal* (not external) jugular vein by its characteristic pulsation, just above the clavicle.
- Measure or estimate the mean vertical height of the venous pulsation above the manubriosternal angle.

Do not rely on the external jugular venous pressure since this vein is valved and prone to kinking, although if it does not drain after occlusion then it is usually associated with a raised JVP.

The internal jugular pulsation can be exaggerated by pressing gently subcostally on the right (hepatojugular reflux). Again warn the patient that it may be uncomfortable.

If the venous pressure is grossly elevated, pulsation may not be visible, and the distended vein may go unnoticed unless the patient is sat up to 90°. Conversely, if the venous pressure is low, as in shock, the vein may not be visible unless the patient is laid down.

Under special circumstances where continuous monitoring of the venous pressure is indicated (such as circumstances where a large volume of fluid is required to be infused in an acidotic diabetic patient with concomitant ventricular failure), this is done by insertion of a central venous catheter.

Phlebotomy

Learning objectives

1 To be able to venesect a patient with minimum distress to the patient and effort to you.
2 To be able to bottle, label, store and dispatch samples appropriately.
3 To practise SAFELY in this potentially biohazardous area.

Taking blood samples for basic and arcane analyses is seen as the stuff of teaching hospitals. By the time you are foundation doctors you must be an expert in this area.

The key to both effortlessness and safety is being *organised* and methodical. Do not rush about using equipment that isn't appropriate in conditions that are suboptimal. Have everything ready in advance and make sure both you and the patient are comfortable and the lighting, etc., is adequate (i.e. not leaning over the 'cot-sides', using a tattered tourniquet in the pitch dark). Universal precautions regarding risk of infection are essential, as is hand hygiene.

Remember that certain tests require patients' consent and counselling. Make sure that you are NOT being asked to do this kind of case.

Equipment

- clinically clean tray or receiver
- tourniquet
- syringe(s) of appropriate size or vacutainer
- 21 swg needle (green)
- swab saturated with isopropyl alcohol 70%
- sterile cotton wool balls
- sterile adhesive plaster or hypo-allergenic tape
- labelled blood specimen bottle(s)
- specimen requisition forms

- gloves
- plastic apron
- sharps box
- eye protection if deemed necessary by risk assessment

Procedure

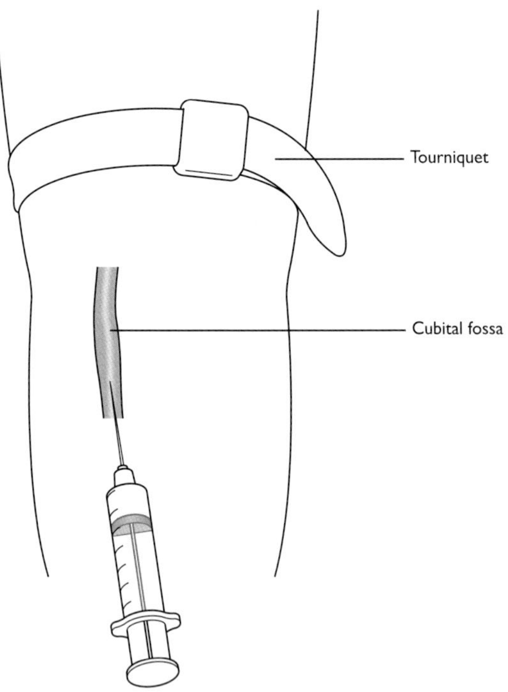

- Approach the patient in a confident manner and explain the procedure to them.
- Allow the patient to ask questions and discuss any preferences and problems that have arisen previously.
- Wash hands using liquid soap and water or alcohol hand rub, and allow to dry before starting.

- Have all necessary equipment with you at the patient's side.
- Ensure privacy, lighting and access are optimal.
- Support the chosen limb.
- Apply a tourniquet to the upper arm on the chosen side, making sure it does not obstruct arterial flow. The position of the tourniquet may be varied, e.g. if a vein in the hand is to be used it may be placed on the forearm.
- The arm may be placed in a dependent position. The patient may assist by clenching and unclenching the fist.
- The veins may be tapped lightly. A patent full vein can be identified by palpating it proximally with the fingers of one hand while tapping it distally with the fingers of your other hand. A transmitted 'pulse' should be detected.
- If all these measures are unsuccessful, remove the tourniquet and apply moist heat, e.g. a hot compress, soak limb in hot water.
- Select a vein.
- Put on gloves.
- Clean patient's skin carefully for at least 15 seconds using an appropriate preparation and allow to dry. Do not re-palpate the vein or touch the skin.
- Anchor the vein by applying manual traction on the skin a few centimetres below the proposed insertion site.
- Insert the needle smoothly at an angle of approximately 30° while aspirating gently on the syringe plunger. Avoid excessive 'sucking' with the syringe as this will collapse the vein. The shaft of a straight needle may be bent slightly at the hub to enable the entry to be as flush with the skin as possible. If using a vacutainer, once the needle has been inserted under the skin attach the first vacutainer. Always leave the fluoride tube until last as it can interfere with biochemical tests.
- Level off the needle as soon as a flashback of blood is seen in the needle hub.

- Advance the needle approximately 2 mm into the vein, if possible.
- Do not exert any pressure on the needle.
- Withdraw the required amount of blood using a syringe or vacutainer.
- Release the tourniquet. In some instances this may be requested at the beginning of sampling as inaccurate measurements may be caused by haemostasis, e.g. blood calcium levels.
- Pick up a sterile wool ball and place it over the puncture point.
- Do not apply pressure until the needle has been fully removed as this will be painful.
- Pressure should be applied until the bleeding has ceased, approximately one minute. Longer may be required if current disease or treatment interferes with clotting mechanisms. The patient may apply pressure with the finger.
- Where a syringe has been used, transfer the blood to appropriate specimen bottles as soon as possible, making sure that the correct quantity is placed in each container. If you under- or overfill the bottle, the proportion of anticoagulant will be incorrect and this may render the test useless.
- Mix well if the bottle contains an anticoagulant.
- Label the bottles with the relevant details. It is infuriating for you and everyone when the lab refuses to analyse the specimen you sent because it was inadequately labelled.
- Inspect the puncture point before applying a dressing.
- Ascertain whether the patient is allergic to adhesive plaster.
- Apply an adhesive plaster or alternative dressing.
- Ensure that the patient is comfortable
- Discard waste, making sure it is placed in the correct containers, e.g. sharps into designed receptacle.
- Follow hospital procedure for collection of specimens to the laboratory.

- Wash hands.
- Record procedure in patient's notes.

Disposal of sharps and other waste

Learning objectives

1. To understand the chain of responsibility for disposal of waste.
2. To be able to handle and dispose of sharps appropriately.

Hospital clinical areas are potentially dangerous both to staff and patients. It is vital that we all adopt a simple code of practice to minimise risk in the workplace. One moment of sloppy practice could quite easily finish your career before it has started.

- Disposal of clinical waste is the responsibility of the person who generated it. Except in extraordinary circumstances, it is unacceptable for any student or doctor of any level of seniority to leave a trolley of clinical waste or sharps lying around for someone else to clear away.
- Ordinary 'household' type waste (paper, packaging, etc.) is disposed of in black plastic bin liners.
- Clinical waste (e.g. blood and other fluids, wound dressings) is disposed of in yellow bags labelled 'Clinical waste—for incineration'. These are available in all clinical areas.
- Under NO CIRCUMSTANCES must sharps be placed in these bags. 'Sharps' include: needles, blades, glass ampoules, plastic Venflons even without the needle, Seldinger wires.
- 'Sharps' are placed in yellow rigid plastic boxes or buckets, which are always clearly labelled as such.

Key practice points

- Always carry your sharps on a tray or trolley. Never wield them.
- Never hand sharps to anyone else.

- Ideally, take the sharps bin to the place where you intend to carry out your procedure. In this way you can bin them immediately and you won't need to leave them around or transport them.
- Never re-sheath a needle or cannula.
- Never put your hand inside a sharps bin. This sounds totally obvious, but bins are often quite full and so the temptation is to stuff your sharps in it, rather than requesting a new one.

Peripheral venous cannulation

Learning objectives

1 To be able to successfully cannulate a peripheral vein with minimum distress to the patient and effort for you.

2 To describe the indications for, and hazards of, venous cannulation.

You must be expert at this by the time you are a foundation doctor. Learning good technique now will pay dividends.

Equipment

- clinically clean tray
- tourniquet
- IV cannula of appropriate size (Venflons)
- syringe containing saline flush 1 hepflush
- swab saturated with isopropyl alcohol 70%
- sterile adhesive tape or plaster
- sharps box

Procedure

- **Follow the guidelines for hand washing.**
- Approach the patient and explain what you are going to do and why. Listen to any of their concerns. Be sympathetic and reassure them with your confidence.
- Choose a site—try to avoid the antecubital fossa as it can be uncomfortable for the patient and have variable flow. Avoid the dorsum of the hand

unless the cannula is for short-term use, and for low-flow infusions or drugs. The best choice is the cephalic vein, in the forearm. It is large, accessible and any infusion set can be secured out of the way, making it less likely to be pulled out and easily visible.

- Support the limb and apply a tourniquet to the upper arm.
- Select a vein and the device based on vein size and site. Don't use anything smaller than an 18 G cannula for infusion of fluid and blood. 16 G is better.
- Put on gloves.
- Clean the patient's skin with the swab and allow to dry.
- If requested, place a bleb of intradermal lignocaine 1% in the overlying skin or use local anaesthetic cream.
- Anchor the vein (see Phlebotomy) and insert the IV cannula (Venflon) smoothly into the vein at an angle of approximately 30° until a flashback of blood is seen in the hub. Do not dither or hesitate once you have pierced the skin. The longer you dither, the more uncomfortable it is, and unless you approach the vein smartly it is liable to move out of the way if at all mobile.
- On observing the flashback, flatten the angle of the cannula to the skin and carefully advance the whole cannula (needle and sheath) a further 1 mm. If you do not do this, you risk failing to be able to advance the cannula over the needle. If you overdo it, you risk transfixing the vein (i.e. the needle piercing and emerging from the opposite wall of the vein).
- Keep the needle fixed and advance the plastic cannula alone a few millimetres into the vein. At this point the tip of the needle is guarded and the whole assembly can be advanced without risk of transfixing the vein or buckling the cannula.
- Palpate the vein and feel where the tip of the plastic cannula is. Gently press over this site so that

you can remove the needle from the cannula and cap it, without allowing blood to leak out. Pressing over the cannula itself (as opposed to the tip) will not prevent a leak unless you press so hard as to crush it; which is not recommended. No matter how slick your cannulation, you will not look cool or be popular if you allow blood to pour over the bed or dressings.

- Place the sharp directly into the sharps bin at your side.
- Apply the adhesive plaster and tape provided to secure the cannula. A flimsy proprietary paper dressing will not be sufficient to secure a cannula on a sweaty clammy patient. It is very much in your own (as well as the patient's) interest to secure it properly, with a proper cannula dressing (e.g. Vecafix).
- Flush the cannula with saline.
- Ensure that the patient is comfortable. Thank them for their patience.
- Discard waste in the containers provided.
- Wash hands.
- Record procedure in patient's notes and insert a Visual Infusion Phlebitis (VIP) score sticker in the patient chart (see below).

Indications and hazards

Venous cannulation is relatively benign, but indwelling IV devices carry a small risk of hospital acquired infection (MRSA cellulitis, septicaemia, endocarditis) and embolus (thrombus and air), and should not be undertaken unless the potential benefits outweigh these small risks. If the cannula is for administration of fluids or antibiotics, ask yourself if enteral fluids are feasible, or if oral or rectal antibiotics are appropriate. These are also cheaper.

If a cannula site appears inflamed or suppurating, the cannula should be removed and the wound site swabbed. Ask a senior for advice on this.

VIP score (Visual Infusion Phlebitis score)

IV site appears healthy	0	**No signs of phlebitis** OBSERVE CANNULA
One of the following is evident: **slight pain near IV site or slight redness near IV site**	1	**Possible first signs of phlebitis** OBSERVE CANNULA
Two of the following are evident: **pain near IV site; erythema; swelling**	2	**Early stage of phlebitis** RESITE CANNULA
All of the following are evident: **pain along path of cannula; erythema; induration**	3	**Medium stage of phlebitis** RESITE CANNULA CONSIDER TREATMENT
All of the following are evident and extensive: **pain along path of cannula; erythema; induration; palpable venous cord**	4	**Advanced stage of phlebitis or start of thrombophlebitis** RESITE CANNULA CONSIDER TREATMENT
All of the following are evident and extensive: **pain along path of cannula; erythema; induration; palpable venous cord; pyrexia**	5	**Advanced stage of thrombophlebitis** INITIATE TREATMENT RESITE CANNULA

Setting up an IV infusion

Learning objectives

1 To use appropriate devices to infuse a prescribed fluid intravenously.

2 To be able to complete a fluid prescription and fluid balance chart in the standard manner.

3 To connect fluid and analgesic infusions safely with 'anti-reflux valves'.

Equipment

- appropriate fluid bag
- appropriate giving set
- short extension tubing if necessary

  - anti-reflux valve if necessary
  - drip-pole

Procedure

- Explain to the patient what you are doing and why.
- Cannulate a vein in the forearm as described elsewhere. As this cannula will be used for infusion of fluids it is preferable if it is a cephalic vein. If a cannula in the dorsum of the hand is connected to a heavy giving-set (with perhaps a three-way tap in circuit, adding extra leverage) it will be constantly moving and will eventually pull out or work loose.
- Check the fluid prescription chart for:
  - type of fluid
  - volume
  - period over which to be infused.
- With a nurse or senior colleague, check fluid bag concords with prescription. Check that it contains no un-prescibed additions (e.g. potassium).
- Close the wheel clamp on the giving set line.
- With the bag suspended on a pole, pierce the outlet port on the bag with the spike of the giving-set fluid chamber.
- Squeeze the fluid chamber and release. Repeat until the chamber is about half full.
- With the giving-set line below the level of the bag, slowly open the wheel clamp and allow fluid to leave the chamber and purge the line of air. Don't do this too quickly or air bubbles will be forced from the chamber down the line. When the line is completely purged of air, close the wheel clamp.
- Remove the cap from the cannula (with your finger pressing on the tip of the cannula within the vein to prevent spillage) and firmly screw the giving-set connector. If the site of the cannula is such that the direct application of the giving-set makes it unwieldy, or the weight of the giving-set

is transmitted directly to the cannula, use a short, lightweight extension piece (a few inches long) to allow a safer connection.

- Tape the giving-set tubing to the arm and make sure there are no potential snags with pyjamas or bedding. Do not tape the tubing in such a way as to lever the cannula at its insertion site.
- Check that the drip runs freely when fully opened, then adjust the drip rate according to the prescription. With a standard set, one drop per second will infuse a litre of saline in about 6 hours.
- Make entry in notes and in fluid chart. Note starting time. Sign legibly.

Anti-reflux valves

Many surgical patients receive analgesia from a Patient Controlled Analgesia (PCA) device. This is a morphine infusion which is actuated by the patient on demand. You will not be expected to set up such a device, but you might be involved in administering fluids to such patients. If the PCA and fluid infusion share a common cannula (via a three-way tap or Y-piece connector) there is a potential for harm to the patient as follows. If the vein becomes occluded the gravity-fed drip will stop running. However, the morphine infusion pump will continue to deliver morphine. This cannot gain access to the patient because the cannula is occluded so instead it is pumped retrogradely up the fluid giving-set. If the cannula were then to be unblocked, either spontaneously or by flushing, the drip would start to run and would carry the large dose of morphine (accumulated in the giving-set over several hours) into the patient as a bolus. This may cause respiratory arrest.

This is prevented by using an anti-reflux valve (Cardiff valve). This is a Y-piece connector, one of whose limbs is valved. It is vital to get the connection right. Fluid is connected to the valved limb and drug is connected to the unvalved limb.

Arterial blood gas sampling

Learning objectives

1 To be able to locate, immobilise and puncture an appropriate artery with minimum distress to the patient and minimum effort for you.
2 How to treat the blood sample so as to minimise artefact in analysis.

Arterial sampling is rarely done in stable patients or in the outpatient setting. Almost by definition, these patients may be sick; with respiratory, circulatory or metabolic disturbances. They may be anxious and frightened. The high quality of your communication with them is doubly important.

Equipment

- clinically clean tray
- swab saturated with isopropyl alcohol 70%
- cotton wool balls 1
- gauze swabs
- sterile adhesive tape
- 2 ml syringe containing 0.1 ml heparin (1000 iu/ml)
- 23 swg needle (blue hub)
- cap and label for syringe
- gloves and sharps bin

Procedure

- Explain what you are going to do and why.
- Allow the patient to ask questions and discuss any preferences as appropriate.
- Assemble appropriate equipment.
- Follow the guidelines for handwashing.
- Choose the most appropriate site.
  - Radial artery—palpate just lateral to flexor carpi radialis at the wrist.
  - Brachial artery—palpate just medial to the bicipital aponeurosis in the antecubital fossa.
  - Femoral artery—palpate just below the inguinal ligament at its mid-point.
- The radial artery is usually the most appropriate, and is easily punctured in a stable patient. If the radial

pulse is weak then the brachial is an alternative. The median nerve lies in close relation to the artery at the level of the antecubital fossa so if you are unsuccessful in locating the artery, there is no place for continued 'stabbings' in the vicinity. Move on to another site. The femoral artery is large and usually foolproof. This is a less dignified site in the conscious patient and the area is generally less clean. Beware patients with peripheral vascular disease who may have atheromatous plaques in the femoral artery. These may break off and embolise ('trash') the limb. Be aware also that the femoral nerve lies 1 cm lateral to the artery.

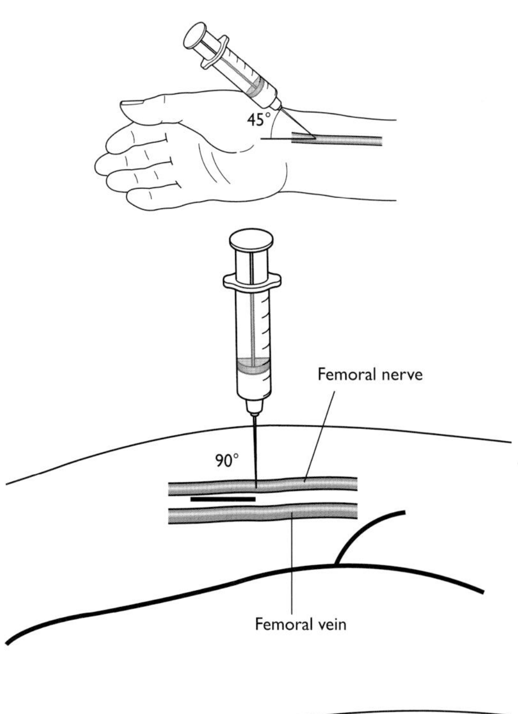

- Support the limb.
- Put on gloves.
- Clean the patient's skin with the swab and allow to dry.
- Inject an intradermal bleb of local anaesthetic using 25 swg needle and 1% lignocaine.
- With your palpating index finger over the artery, insert the needle at the point of maximum pulsation at 45° to skin and advance until pulsatile blood is seen filling the syringe.
- Once required volume is collected remove needle smoothly, while applying firm pressure to the site with cotton wool or gauze.
- Maintain pressure for 3 minutes or until there is no further bleeding
- Apply the adhesive tape.
- Expel air from the syringe and seal it with cap.
- Dispose of needle in sharps bin by your side and label syringe.
- Remove gloves and discard.
- Thank the patient for their co-operation
- Dispatch sample as soon as possible.

Handling of arterial samples

- Expel air from the syringe as soon as possible. If the sample is allowed to equilibrate with a large volume of room air, the measured blood gas values will tend to a POa of 20 KPa and PCO_2 of zero.
- Never use a larger volume of heparin than 0.1 ml of 1000 u/ml (i.e. just enough to 'wet' the hub of the needle). Heparin is acidic and will give an artefactual metabolic acidosis if added in excess.
- Blood is living tissue. Oxygen continues to be consumed in the syringe in transit. Do not allow it to stand around for more than 10 minutes before analysis. If delay is inevitable, put the sample on ice.

Passing a urinary catheter

Learning objectives

1 To be confident and competent to catheterise the bladder safely with minimum distress to the patient.

2 To be aware of the anatomical abnormalities that may have led to urinary retention and how these may impact on the procedure.

3 To be able to formulate a plan in the event of failure to catheterise the bladder.

Equipment

- clean procedure trolley with 'catheter pack' or similar
- selection of sizes of Foley catheter (from 12 to 16 French)
- Savlon-type skin prep (NOT iodine, NOT spirit)
- saline and 10 ml syringe to fill balloon
- topical lignocaine gel

Procedure: male

- Introduce yourself. Explain what you are going to do and why. Listen to the patient's concerns.
- Wash and dry hands.
- Wearing sterile gloves, place sterile towels across the patient's thighs and under buttocks.
- Place a collecting vessel for urine between the patient's legs.
- Wrap a sterile swab around the penis and use this to hold the shaft without contaminating your gloves. Retract the foreskin, if necessary, and clean the glans penis with saline or antiseptic (Savlon-type) solution.
- Instil all the 10 ml of 2% lignocaine gel into the urethra to achieve topical anaesthesia.
- Hold the urethral meatus of the glans penis firmly closed to prevent the gel being released and wipe the underside of the penile shaft in a downward direction several times with a dry swab to move the gel towards the prostatic urethra. Wait 2–3 minutes for the anaesthetic to work.

- Grasp the shaft of penis with the non-dominant hand, raising it until totally extended.
- Hold the catheter in the dominant hand and gently pass it into the urethral meatus. Continue slowly and smoothly to pass the catheter through the urethra into the bladder. If resistance is felt at the prosthetic urethra/sphincter region, ask the patient to relax the muscle as if he were going to void urine or cough.
- Once the urine starts to flow, pass the catheter a further 5 cm to ensure balloon is in the bladder before slowly inflating the balloon with 10 ml of sterile water or saline.
- Pull the catheter gently. It should withdraw a few centimetres until the balloon prevents further egress.
- Attach catheter to appropriate draining system and tape catheter laterally to thigh.
- Ensure that the glans penis is clean and then reduce and reposition the foreskin.
- Make sure patient is comfortable and thank them for their co-operation.
- Dispose of waste materials in yellow clinical waste bag.
- Wash hands.
- Record procedure in patient's notes.

Procedure: female

- Introduce yourself and explain what you are going to do and why.
- Wearing *double* sterile gloves, place sterile towels across the patient's thighs and under the buttocks.
- Place a collecting vessel for urine between the patient's legs.
- Separate the labia minora so that the urethral meatus is seen. Using non-lint gauze swabs, one hand should be used to maintain labial separation until catheterisation is completed.
- Clean around the urethral orifice with normal saline or an antiseptic solution, using single downward strokes, discarding the swab after each stroke.

- Discard outer gloves.
- Lubricate the catheter with a sterile anaesthetic lubricating jelly.
- Introduce the tip of the catheter into the urethral orifice in an upward and backward direction.
- Advance the catheter until 5–6 cm have been inserted.
- Advance the catheter 6–8 cm.
- Inflate the balloon according to the manufacturer's instructions, having ensured that the catheter is draining adequately.
- Withdraw the catheter slightly and connect it to the drainage system.
- Tape the catheter and drainage system to the thigh.
- Make the patient comfortable and ensure that the area is dry.
- Thank the patient for their co-operation.
- Dispose of equipment in a disposable plastic bag.
- Make an entry in the notes detailing the procedure.

Checkpoints

Male: If it is not possible to advance the catheter up the urethra, do not force it. Try a smaller size or stiffer catheter. Re-orientate the penile shaft and try again. If it is still impossible, specialist assistance may be required. If catherisation is a matter of urgency in an obstructed patient, and attempts *per urethram* have failed, you should consider and plan for (but not attempt yourself) a percutaneous suprapubic catheterisation.

Female: In a large patient, it may be difficult to separate the legs and labia and hold the catheter single-handedly. Request assistance to act as another pair of hands to part the labia.

It is important not to inflate the balloon unless you are sure it is well inside the bladder and not inside the urethra. Once inflated, ability to withdraw the catheter a few centimetres before it comes to a halt confirms that the balloon is correctly positioned. If you cannot do this, deflate the balloon and reposition.

Bladder emptying: Rapid emptying of a chronically distended and obstructed bladder may cause autonomic disturbance and may even disrupt the bladder epithelium causing haematuria. Consequently, in these circumstances the bladder should be drained slowly and in stages.

Lumbar puncture

Learning objectives

1 To be able to describe the indications and contra-indications for lumbar puncture.
2 To be able to describe the risks associated with the procedure and how they relate to the potential diagnostic benefits, so that the student may reasonably be able to obtain informed consent for the procedure.
3 To know the equipment required.
4 To be able to perform the procedure on a manikin.

Equipment

- sterile lumbar puncture procedure pack
  - lumbar puncture needle (atraumatic type)
  - manometer
  - swabs, gallipots, towels, cleaning fluid
- local anaesthetic, syringes, skin infiltration needles
- sterile containers for CSF samples (at least 3)

Procedure

- Introduce yourself and explain the procedure to the patient. Either you or a senior colleague will have obtained informed consent beforehand. Check the details are correct.
- Position the patient with lumbar spine flexed, in the left lateral position with the knees pulled up into the chest and the head tucked down to the chest.
- Identify the third and fourth lumbar spines. These are close to the line running between the iliac crests. Mark the chosen space with pen.
- Wash hands and put on gown, mask and gloves.

- Prepare equipment using aseptic technique.
- Clean with chlorhexidine or iodine and drape the area.
- Infiltrate the skin and soft tissues with local anaesthetic.
- Advance lumbar puncture needle through the spinal ligaments. If the spinal flexion is optimal the needle will be perpendicular to the skin in all planes. Often, however, it requires to be angulated slightly cephalad.
- Once the tip of the needle pierces the dura a slight 'give' will be felt. Withdraw stilette and allow a few drops of CSF to escape.
- 'Opening pressure' can be measured using the manometer.
- CSF samples can be collected serially in the sterile containers and labelled 1st, 2nd, 3rd, etc.
- Remove the needle and apply dressing.
- Dispose of all sharps in the sharps box.
- Remove gloves and wash hands.
- Thank the patient for their co-operation.

Lumbar puncture is a procedure with a very low risk of serious morbidity.

Indications for diagnostic LP

- Suspected subarachnoid haemorrhage
- Suspected meningitis/encephalitis
- Suspected haematological malignancy

Contraindications to LP

- Raised intracranial pressure with dilated ventricles
- Anticoagulated patient (relative)

Complications

The commonest complication of this procedure is a severe 'post-dural puncture headache' (PDPH). It occurs with a frequency of about 1% and is related to continued leakage of CSF from the subarachnoid space. PDPH is much more likely to occur if 'cutting' type needles are used (e.g. Yale, Quincke). The most appropriate needle is an 'atraumatic' non-cutting type (Whitacre or Sprotte). The smallest size that can be handled should be used (25 gauge is ideal).

PDPH can be severe and disabling. It may also confuse the clinical picture of the initial clinical presentation. Very rarely it can cause subarachnoid haemorrhage and isolated cranial nerve palsies. It should be treated in the first instance with fluid rehydration and simple analgesics, and referred to a specialist (anaesthetist) with experience in treating this condition.

Infection and meningitis are rare but recognised complications of the procedure.

Aseptic technique and hand washing

Learning objective

1 To know and be able to demonstrate a simple and effective drill for carrying out routine surgical procedures 'aseptically'.

Procedure

- Explain procedure to patient and request their co-operation in helping keeping the sterile field clear.
- Organise an assistant to help you, i.e. to pass various items when you are 'scrubbed'. Arrange this now, otherwise there may be no help available when you need it.
- Wear protective clothing such as visor and apron if appropriate.
- Wash hands with liquid soap and dry with paper towel.
- Arrange sterile pack (for whatever procedure) on a procedure trolley. Ensure pack is sterile and open using corners of the pack. Open a packet of gloves and place it on the pack.
- Wash hands again using Hibiscrub or similar antibacterial. Hold hand upright and dry with a sterile paper towel, with a single downward wipe for each arm.

- Don a gown if appropriate.
- Glove each hand.
- Using forceps in the pack arrange sterile field with handles of the instruments in one corner.
- Carry out procedures.
- Avoid contamination by using a 'no-touch' technique. Use forceps to pick up and manipulate 'dirty' objects. Use 'swabs on sticks' (as opposed to holding swabs in your hand) to clean patient's skin, etc., and discard into a waste bag after a single use. Do not put them back on the trolley in your clean field.
- Dispose of waste in yellow bag
- Declare in the notes that an 'aseptic technique' was used.

Passing a nasogastric tube

Learning objectives

1 To be able to pass a nasogastric tube in a fellow student and a patient quickly and effectively, causing minimum distress to the subject.

2 To be able to assess the position of the tube after insertion with confidence and to write the details of the procedure concisely in the notes.

Procedure

- Introduce yourself and explain what you are going to do and why.
- Prepare the 'patient'. Make sure that the 'patient' is sitting comfortably and that they know what is expected of them during the procedure.
- Establish if there is any past history of trauma/surgery to either nostril or previous difficulties in passing a nasogastric tube which will alert you to potential problems.
- Slightly extend the neck so that the nostrils are easier to access.
- Prepare the tube. Lubricate the tube with water-soluble jelly (K-Y or similar). Be careful not to occlude the end of the tube with a blob of jelly, but make

sure the lower third of the tube is well lubricated and not just the tip.

- Gently insert the tube into the chosen nostril and slide along the floor of the nose. Make sure that any curve in the tube is kept pointing downwards rather than side to side or upwards.
- When the patient feels the tube in the back of their throat, **stop**.

Tips

- Advance the tube slowly—let the patient get used to the sensation.
- If the tube won't slide easily, don't push hard. The nostril is probably obstructed. Stop and try the other side.

Getting the tube into the oesophagus

- With the tube in the top of the oropharynx, gently flex the neck to make the angle between nasopharynx and oropharynx more acute. This helps to steer the tube down the back of the oropharynx and not forward into the mouth. The action is a slow deliberate one. Pushing is only likely to make the patient gag and draw the tube into the mouth.
- Ask the patient to swallow several times as you advance the tube. As the upper oesophageal sphincter relaxes, you should feel the tube slide down into the oesophagus freely.

Tips

- Try to co-ordinate the advance of the tube with the swallowing actions.
- Have the patient sip a glass of water if they find it difficult to swallow spontaneously.
- If the patient coughs, draw the tube back a little and let them settle again before continuing.
- If the tube keeps bending forward (worse with small tubes) try stiffening the end by cooling it in iced water before starting again. (However, this can

make the passage through the nose slightly more uncomfortable.)

Passing the tube down the oesophagus

- Once through the upper sphincter, the tube should slide easily down the oesophagus.
- Swallowing during this also helps the tube to advance.
- If there is any significant resistance to the passage of the tube, stop.
- Check that you are not already in the stomach and have miscalculated (see below).
- If the tube is still in the oesophagus and will not advance, stop and remove the tube. Do not try to force the passage.

Checking the position of the tube

The tube has graduations on the side to help you judge distance. Remember the average distance from incisors to the OG junction in an adult is around 60 cm. There are two ways to check that the tube is in the stomach.

1. Inject air down the tube with a syringe and auscultate over the stomach. You should hear the tube bubbling.
2. Aspirate the tube. If liquid is returned then you are probably in the stomach. To be sure you can test the fluid with litmus paper to check that it is acid. The tube is usually secured in position with a surgical tape to the side of the face.

Tips

Bile staining of the fluid does not necessarily mean that the tube has passed through the pylorus into the duodenum. A number of people reflux bile into the stomach 'normally'.

Common problems with a nasogastric tube

- Irritation and even ulceration of the nares where the tube exits. This can be distressing for the patient and needs good nursing care to prevent it happening when the tube is present for any length of time.

- Irritation of the pharynx (worse with larger tubes). Can be improved by sucking ice cubes or anaesthetic lozenges.
- Epistaxis (usually your fault—bad technique causing trauma to the nasal epithelium). Take the tube out and leave the insertion to another time.

Administration of IV drugs

Learning objectives

1 To be able to interpret, check and make an entry in a drug prescription chart.
2 To be confident and competent in IV drug administration according to a standard protocol.
3 To be aware of, and able to deal with, any possible immediate complications of IV drug administration.

Until recently most or all IV drugs were administered by doctors, most of whom did so without specific training, and sometimes badly. Today, most IV drugs administered on the wards are done so by nurses who have received training and do it well. This skill station sets out a simple standard protocol that ensures safety.

- Consult the patient's prescription sheet, and ascertain the following:
  - drug
  - dose
  - date and time of administration
  - route and method of administration
  - diluent as appropriate
  - validity of prescription
  - signature of doctor.
- If you suspect an error you should seek to clarify the details with the prescriber. Consultation with a pharmacist or the BNF may be advisable. As a doctor and the administrator of the drug, you share responsibility with the prescriber for the consequences of any gross error.
- Collect and check all equipment.
- Check that the packaging of all equipment is intact and in date.

- Wash hands with liquid soap followed by alcohol hand rub.
- Prepare needle(s), syringe(s), etc., on a tray or receiver.
- Inspect all equipment.
- Select the drug in the appropriate size or dosage and check the expiry date.
- Proceed with the preparation of the drug, using protective clothing if advisable.

Single dose ampoule: solution

- Inspect the solution for cloudiness or particulate matter. If this is present, discard and follow hospital guidelines on what action to take, e.g. return drug to pharmacy.
- Tap the neck of the ampoule gently to knock down any solution in it.
- Cover the neck of the ampoule with a sterile swab and snap it open.
- Inspect the solution for glass fragments; if present, discard.
- Withdraw the required amount of solution, tilting the ampoule if necessary.
- Hold the syringe spout uppermost and tap it to dislodge any air bubbles. Expel air.
- Remove the needle using a safety device, for example mushroom device.
- Dispose of needle in sharps box.
- Apply new sheathed needle or cap.

Single dose ampoule: powder

- Tap the neck of the ampoule gently.
- Cover the neck of the diluent ampoule with a swab and snap it open. If the diluent is not provided with the drug, check what it is supposed to be by referring to the data sheet in the packaging. If water is required, use water. Saline and water are NOT interchangeable.
- Add the correct diluent with syringe and needle carefully down the wall of the ampoule.

- Agitate the ampoule and inspect the contents.
- When the solution is clear, withdraw the prescribed amount as follows. Fill the syringe (used to inject the diluent) with air of the same volume. Invert the ampoule containing the drug solution and hold in your non-dominant hand. Pierce the rubber seal with the needle mounted on the air-filled syringe held in your dominant hand. Slowly inject a few ml of air and then aspirate the same few ml of drug solution back, keeping the tip of the needle below the water line at all times. Repeat this procedure until all the drug is aspirated.
- Leave the needle in the rubber bung, inserted to the hilt.
- Dispose of ampoule and needle in sharps box
- Apply new sheathed needle or cap.

Administration to patient

- Introduce yourself to the patient and check their ID with the drug prescription.
- Double check any allergies.
- Explain what you are going to do and why.
- Have all your equipment available on a clean tray or receiver.
- Check the site and patency of the IV cannula, and flush it with saline.
- Inject the drug at a rate determined by the data sheet instructions. For most antibiotics this is a rate of about 5 ml every 30 seconds. There are some notable exceptions such as erythromicin. Do not add drugs to the *in situ* drip bag. This is very bad practice for a number of reasons. Other drugs such as amiodarone, ranitidine, aminophylline may need to be given by infusion rather than injection.
- A slow administration allows time for you to assess any immediate adverse effects such as local pain or anaphylaxis, and to stop administration sooner than you otherwise could.

- Flush the cannula with saline to remove traces of drug from the hub and to prevent phlebitis.
- Dispose of sharps in sharps box, and syringes in clinical waste bags.
- Make entry in drug chart stating drug, dose, route of admin, time and date. Sign it legibly and append your bleep number.

Administration of drugs by continuous infusion

Learning objectives

1 To be able to interpret, check and make an entry in a drug prescription chart.
2 To be confident and competent in the use of infusion devices.
3 To be aware of, and able to deal with, any possible immediate complications of IV drug administration.

Drugs administered by IV infusion fall usually into one of three categories:

- drugs that are irritant (cause phlebitis) and so cannot be administered as a bolus
- drugs that have a short half-life (heparin, insulin)
- drugs that are very potent (adrenaline, noradrenaline, etc.).

Make sure you know which of these you are dealing with.

Equipment

- clinically clean receiver or tray containing the prepared drug to be administered
- patient's prescription chart
- recording sheet or book as required by law or hospital policy
- protective clothing as required by hospital policy
- container of appropriate intravenous infusion fluid
- swab saturated with isopropyl alcohol 70%
- drug additive label

Procedure

- Explain the procedure to the patient.
- Inspect the infusion.
- Wash hands with liquid soap and water and use alcohol hand rub. Allow to dry, and assemble the necessary equipment.
- Check name, strength and volume of intravenous fluid against the prescription chart.
- Check the expiry date of the fluid.
- Check that the packaging is intact.
- Inspect the container and contents in a good light for cracks, punctures, air bubbles, discolouration, haziness and crystalline or particulate matter.
- Check the identity and amount of drug to be added. Consider:
  - compatibility of fluid and additive
  - stability of mixture over the prescription time
  - any special directions for dilution, e.g. pH optimum concentration, etc.
  - sensitivity to external factors such as light
  - any anticipated allergic reaction.
- If any doubts exist about the listed points, consult the pharmacist or BNF/datasheet.
- Any additions must be made immediately before use.
- Wash hands thoroughly using liquid soap and water, dry and then apply alcohol hand rub and allow to dry.
- Expose the injection site on the container by removing any seal present.
- Clean the site with the swab and allow it to dry.
- Inject the drug using a new sterile needle into the bag or bottle.
- Invert the container a number of times, especially if adding to a flexible infusion bag.
- Check again for haziness, discolouration, etc. This can occur even if the mixture is theoretically compatible, thus making vigilance essential.

- Complete the drug additive label and fix it on the bag or bottle. Complete the patient's recording chart and other hospital and/or legally required documents.
- Place the container in a clinically clean receptacle. Wash hands and proceed to the patient.
- Check again that the infusion is running well and that the contents of the previous container have been delivered.
- Switch off the infusion and hang the new container quickly using a no-touch technique.
- Restart the infusion and adjust the rate of flow as prescribed.
- Ask the patient if any abnormal sensations, etc., are experienced.
- Discard waste, sharps into sharps box and other clinical waste into the yellow clinical waste bag.

Mechanical administration of drugs/fluids via a pump or syringe driver may be necessary.

Drug infusion can be administered by a variety of devices. The simplest is drug added to a bag of saline and delivered by gravity-fed burette system. The beauty of this device is its simplicity. However, the flow rate is variable since it is governed by gravity and the resistances within the line and cannula, so vigilance is required.

A variant on this is the IVAC type of pump which has a giving-set that is manipulated by a peristaltic pump. These pumps often have complicated un-intuitive menus, are very sensitive to 'air in the line' and frequently malfunction. You need a lot of patience to use this kind of device. If you can't avoid using one, then ask someone who is thoroughly familiar with it (i.e. the patient's nurse) to show you how to tame it.

Smaller volume infusions are administered with syringe pumps. These are usually simple, have intuitive menus and are more or less foolproof.

Remember to use an anti-reflux valve if the drug infusion is sharing a cannula with an ordinary IV fluid infusion.

Blood glucose analysis and urinalysis

Learning objectives

1 To obtain a small sample of capillary blood with minimum distress to the patient.
2 To use proprietary blood glucose and urine assay kits correctly and obtain results free of artefact.

Blood glucose (using BM 144 test strips)

- Introduce yourself to the patient and explain what you are going to do and why.
- Wash and dry hands thoroughly.
- Use gloves and apron when handling body fluids.
- Remove test strip from container ensuring they are within the appropriate date. Replace the cap on the container to ensure moisture doesn't enter the tube.
- Wipe the patient's finger to remove any glucose that may be present.
- Take sterile lancet. Prick the side of the fingertip. Squeeze finger to obtain large, suspended drop of blood.
- Apply blood to cover both test pads. Do not spread or smear blood. Start timing—EXACTLY 60 SECONDS.
- Hold strip against clean surface. Wipe away blood with fresh cotton wool. Do not use paper which may contain sugars, or the bed clothes. Wipe twice more with clean area of cotton wool. Start timing, again EXACTLY 60 SECONDS.
- Compare strip with colour blocks on tube (colours remain stable for ample reading or checking time). If UPPER pad remains a BUFF colour, the blood glucose level is below 9 mmol/1. Compare LOWER (blue) colour block on the tube to read blood glucose level.
- If UPPER pad changes to GREEN, the blood glucose level is above 9 mmol/1. Therefore the UPPER (green)

pad needs to be compared with the UPPER (green) block on the tube to read the blood glucose level

- If the result is above 17 mmol/1 after 2 minutes, the reaction is not complete. Wait a further 60 seconds. Read again, using only the UPPER (green) block on the tube.
- Interpret results and take action if required.
- Remove gloves and wash hands.
- Record the result where appropriate.

Electrochemical devices are now superseding this pigment-based assay. Here, blood is dropped in a similar way on to an electrode strip containing glucose oxidase enzyme. The resultant redox reaction results in a flow of electrons through the electrode. The magnitude of the current is proportional to the glucose concentration. In true 'plug 'n' play' tradition, these devices are very intuitive and have simple instructions printed on the device.

Measurement of peak flow and vitalography

Learning objectives

1 To understand and be able to describe the utility of measuring peak flow.
2 To be able to measure peak flow reliably and reproducibly.
3 To understand and be able to describe the utility of 'vitalography'.
4 To be able to record a 'vitalograph' reliably and reproducibly.
5 To be able to infer the presence of disease states from your findings.

Measurement of peak flow is a very commonly performed procedure in emergency medicine and the chest clinic. It provides indirect information about airways resistance and is a useful guide to the severity of acute asthma or the monitoring of chronic stable asthma. One of the problems with the validity of measurements like this is that the value obtained is as much dependent on the degree of patient effort and motivation as it is on the airways resistance. For this reason the technique of the supervising clinician is important.

Peak flow

- Approach the patient, introduce yourself and explain what you are about to do and why.
- Select a peak flow meter and ensure that it has a clean cardboard mouthpiece and is 'zeroed'.
- Ask the patient to sit as upright as possible and explain that you would like them to take as big a breath as possible, place their lips tightly around the mouthpiece and blow out as hard and fast as possible. You may wish to demonstrate the action, either with or without actually blowing into the meter (if you do, be sure to replace the mouthpiece).
- Encourage the patient as they are taking a breath in. *Enthusiastically* encourage them to blow out as hard as possible. If you encourage them in a the slow, calm and reserved manner in which you would normally practise medicine you will be rewarded only with a slow, calm and half-hearted effort.
- Aim to make three measurements and record the best of these.

Vitalography

Peak flow measures the maximum flow rate at any time in expiration, regardless of how transiently the flow rate pertains. In chronic obstructive airways disease (COAD) with dynamic airway compression, expiratory flow rate may be moderately high early in expiration, but only for a few milliseconds. The maximum flow rate is therefore not representative of the overall flow rate. In these circumstances, the average flow rate over the first second (FEV1), measured by vitalography, is a more representative figure. The ratio of FEV1 to forced vital capacity (FVC) is a useful discriminator between obstructive and restrictive lung disease.

- Prepare yourself and the patient as above.
- Mount vitalograph paper in the machine and orientate it such that the stylus overlies the zero-time, zero-volume origin.
- Make sure the vitalograph is plugged in.
- Enthusiastically encourage the patient to take the deepest possible breath and blow out as fast as possible, and for as long as possible.
- If possible repeat the measurement three times on the same chart.
- Label the chart with the patient's name and the date.

Setting up oxygen delivery devices

Learning objectives

1 To know the clinical indications and contraindications, including examples, for increasing the inspired oxygen concentration to high levels.

2 To describe simple devices capable of providing high inspired concentration of oxygen, and demonstrate how to set them up.

3 To know the clinical indications, including examples, for increasing the inspired oxygen concentration to **specific predetermined** levels.

4 To describe simple devices capable of providing preset oxygen concentations, and demonstrate how to set them up.

The Hudson mask (variable performance mask)

This is a simple clear plastic mask which is held in place by elastic and through which oxygen flows at a rate set by a 'rotameter' (bobbin flow meter) on the oxygen outlet. The actual concentration of oxygen the patient receives is variable. If the flow rate is set high (e.g. 15 l/min) the effective concentration will be high (say, up to 80%). Even with an oxygen flow rate of 15 l/min, this is still lower than the patient's peak inspiratory flow rate, so some air will be entrained through and around the mask during inspiration, thus diluting the inspired oxygen. The higher the patient's minute volume (and peak inspiratory flow) the greater the dilution. Patients with very shallow respiration (and low peak inspiratory flow) may not entrain any air at all and so may have an inspired oxygen concentration of 100% even with low oxygen flow rates. Such a patient may therefore remain pink (with SpO_2 of 100%) even though they are virtually apnoeic. For this reason, pulse oximeters are not useful monitors of ventilator function in these circumstances.

The indication for these devices is to provide moderate to high concentrations of oxygen in circumstances where the actual value is not critical. They are not suitable for situations where the actual value of FIO_2 is critical.

The HAFOE mask (Venturi or fixed performance mask)

This superficially resembles the Hudson mask. The difference lies in the Venturi device through which the oxygen flows as it enters the mask. The Venturi device is colour-coded for different required oxygen concentrations. Unlike the Hudson mask, the Venturi mask provides a constant and fixed FIO_2 regardless of how the patient breathes. This is achieved by passing a moderate flow of oxygen, say 6 l/min into the Venturi (the actual required flow rate is printed on the device). The Venturi then entrains air into the device at a fixed ratio. If it sucks in air at say 5 volumes per volume of oxygen, then the total flow rate into the mask will be 36 l/min and the oxygen concentration of this mixture will be 34%. The flow rate is so high that it is unlikely that the patient's inspiratory flow rate will exceed it, so no matter how the patient breathes, the inspired oxygen concentration will be constant. Any excess gas escapes around the mask.

Giving an intramuscular injection

Learning objectives

1 To check and prepare the prescribed drug.
2 List all appropriate sites for IM injection.
3 To describe the relevant anatomy of the gluteal region and course of the sciatic nerve.

Intramuscular drugs are most frequently administered by nursing staff. You will occasionally be required to perform this task and must know how to practise safely, avoiding the pitfalls. Bad technique in this procedure, through inadequate (or absent) training, is commonly cited by the medical defence organisations as a frequent cause of doctors being sued.

- Introduce yourself to the patient and explain what you wish to do and why, reassuring them.
- Check the drug prescription and any ALLERGIES.
- Assemble all the things you will need and place on a clean tray.
- Wash your hands and wear gloves.
- Check the vial contents, dose and expiry date.
- Open vial safely and draw diluent and reconstitute drug if necessary.
- Mark the upper outer quadrant of the buttock, if this is the site you choose.
- Clean skin with alcohol swab.
- With 23 g needle (blue) enter this quadrant smartly, perpendicular in all planes, and to a depth of 2–3 cm.
- Ask the patient how they feel (they should tell you if you've winged the sciatic nerve).
- Withdraw the plunger to ensure you are not intravenous and inject slowly. Rapid injection will produce a painful local pressure effect.
- Swab on removal.
- Apply dressing (Elastoplast) centred on puncture mark.
- Dispose of sharps safely.
- Sign the prescription chart.
- Thank the patient for their co-operation.

Ophthalmoscopy

Learning objectives

1 To be able to handle an ophthalmoscope and conduct an examination confidently.
2 To describe the purpose and functions of the instrument.
3 To be able to follow a system for identifying the optic disc, the retina and retinal vessels.

Procedure

- Greet the patient, introduce yourself and explain what you are going to do and why.
- Ensure that the patient is sitting comfortably.
- Dilate the pupils.
- Ask the patient to fixate on a distant object.
- Switch on the ophthalmoscope.
- Set the internal lens setting in the ophthalmoscope to 0.
- Use your right eye to examine the patient's right eye.
- Look through the ophthalmoscope at arm's distance from the patient and observe the right red reflex with your right eye.
- Keep both eyes open if possible.
- Bend forward to approach the patient following the red reflex. Keep the ophthalmoscope upright relative to the patient.
- Locate a retinal blood vessel. You should now be about 10 cm from the patient.
- Adjust the internal lens settings on the ophthalmoscope to bring the retinal vessel into focus.
- Track the vessel towards the optic disc.
- Examine the optic disc, paying particular attention to the colour, cup, vasculature and edge.
- Repeat with the left eye.
- Thank the patient.

Otoscopy

Learning objectives

1 To be able to handle an otoscope and conduct an examination confidently.
2 To describe the purpose and functions of the instrument.

3 To be able to describe the condition of the pinna, postaural area, external auditory meatus and tympanic membrane.

Procedure

- Greet the patient, introduce yourself and explain what you are going to do and why.
- Ensure that the patient is sitting comfortably.
- Examine behind the ear for scars indicating previous mastoid surgery.
- Check the light on the otoscope is bright and select an earpiece appropriate to the size of the external auditory meatus (EAM).
- Hold the otoscope (upside down) at 2 o'clock in the right hand for the right ear, 10 o'clock in the left hand for the left ear.
- Gently pull the pinna up and back in adults and down and back in children to straighten out the cartilaginous EAM.
- Insert the otoscope into the EAM observing any pathology at the entrance to the EAM.
- Gently proceed down the EAM until the eardrum is seen. The EAM is angled a little anteriorly and twisting the otoscope backwards may help.
- Continue to observe as the otoscope is removed as pathology missed on the way in may be seen on the way out.
- Thank the patient.

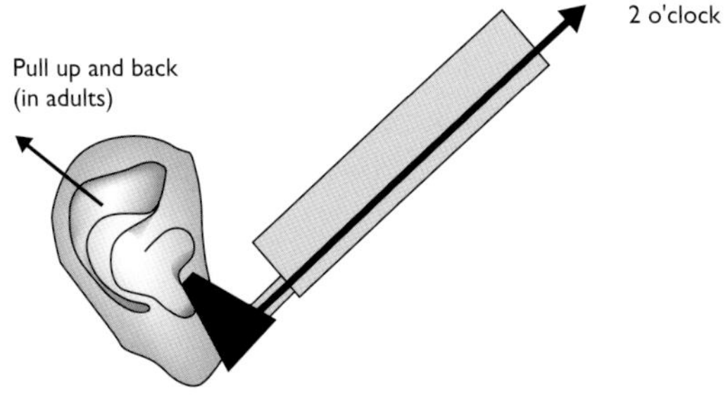

Right ear

Surgical knot tying

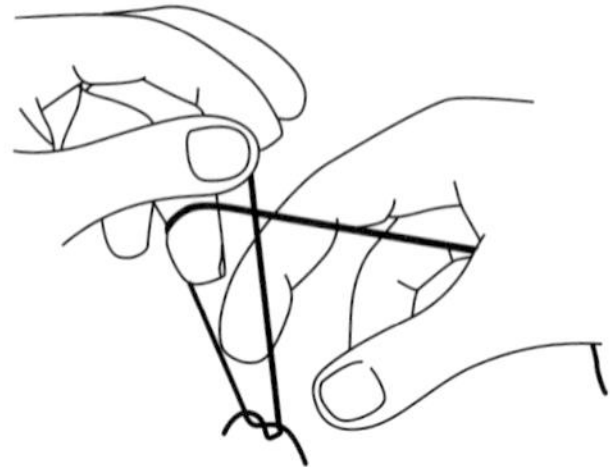

Forming the reverse cross

The left thread is now passed IN FRONT OF the right thread and held in the right hand. The left hand, again, holds the short end and opens up the space between threads while the right thumb and index finger trap the crossing point, this time with the thumb TOWARDS you.

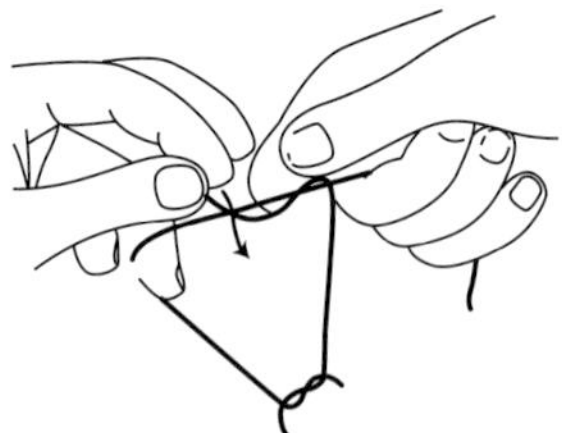

Positioning the thread

The left hand brings the short thread over the 'bar' formed by the long thread and positions it under the control of the right thumb.

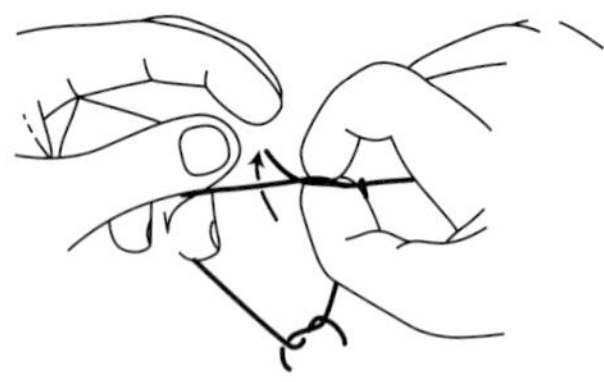

Flipping the thread under

The right hand is now pronated and this flips the thread end under, through the gap between threads.

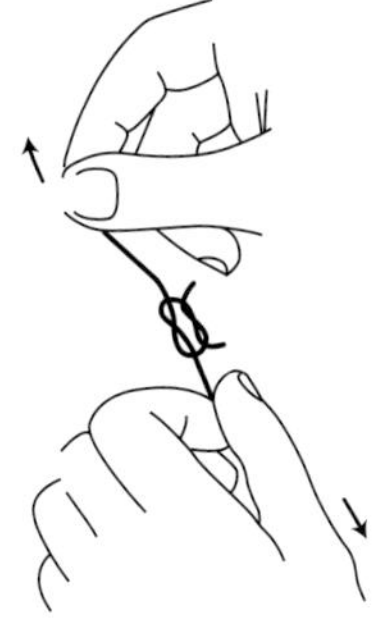

Tying the knot

The left hand picks up the loose end of the thread and pulls it down and towards you to lay the second half of the hitch on top of the first.

Risk assessment for universal precaution

No blood/body fluid contact	No protective clothing
Presence of blood and body fluid and low risk of splashing	Use gloves and apron
Presence of blood and body fluid and high risk of splashing	Use gloves, waterproof gown and eye protection
If uncertain, use protection and assume high risk (Wilson and Breedon, 1990)	

Hand wash techniques

A systemic approach to hand washing and skin disinfection, including applying alcohol rubs, is necessary to ensure all potentially contaminated surfaces are treated.

For example fingertips, between fingers, thumbs, areas of the palms and backs of the hands are frequently missed.

Handwashing process

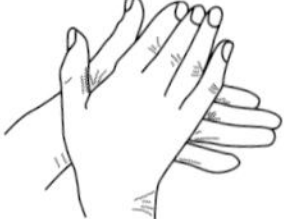

1. run palm to palm

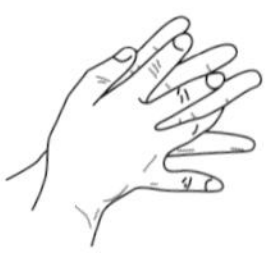

2. right palm over left dorsum and left palm over right dorsum

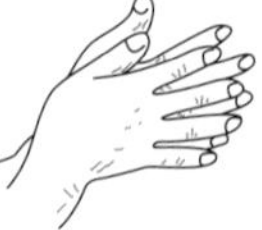

3. palm to palm, fingers interlaced palm over right dorsum

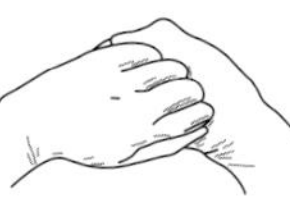

4. backs of fingers to opposing palms back and forwards with fingers interlocked right hand in

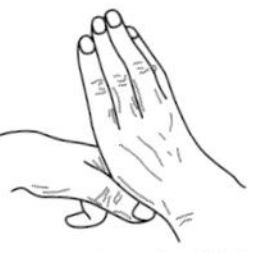

5. rotational rubbing of right thumb clasped in left palm and vice versa

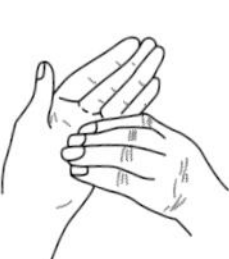

6. rotational rubbing with clasped fingers of left palm and vice versa

This need only take 15–30 seconds.

Hands must be wet before applying the **recommended** amount of soap and rinsed thoroughly before drying. It is important that hands are dried well.

The wrists must be included as part of the hand washing process. This technique normally takes between 15 and 30 seconds.

The same technique is recommended when using alcohol hand rubs but no water is used and the hands and wrists are rubbed until dry. Effective skin disinfection occurs only when the alcohol is rubbed in until the skin is dry; this will ensure adequate contact time.

Handwashing frequency

Hands must be washed after any activity that has contaminated the skin, before food preparation, patient contact or any clinical procedure.

Electronic counting equipment installed on ward hand wash basins has found handwashing frequency

to be much lower than claimed. Guidance on hand contamination and advice on when to wash or disinfect the hands is given in the tables below.

EXAMPLES OF WHEN TO CLEAN THE HANDS

BEFORE	
Aseptic procedures	Entering protective isolation rooms
Surgical procedures and injections	Preparing food
AFTER	
Leaving source isolation rooms	Using the lavatory
Contact with secretions and excretions	Handling bedpans and urine bottles
	Cleaning and making beds

Items and activities ranked according to **EXTENT** of hand contamination

Practices **MORE** likely to contaminate the hands

Direct contact with infected sites

Contact with excretions or secretions from infected patients; contact with excretions or secretions; bedding from infected patient, bed, bath, etc

Moist objects likely to be contaminated—cleaning materials; limited patient contact—taking pulse

Materials in close contact with non-infected patients—bedding, etc.; items not in close contact with patients, e.g. furniture; items never in contact with patients; sterile, disinfected, cleaned materials

Practices **LESS** likely to be associated with hand contamination

HAND WASHING RATIONALE

	SOCIAL HAND WASH	HYGIENIC HAND DISINFECTION	SURGICAL SCRUB
WHY	• To achieve socially clean hands • To remove/destroy transient micro-organisms	• To remove transient micro-organisms	• To remove or destroy all transient micro-organisms, which may also have a prolonged effect • To substantially reduce resident micro-organisms • **A prolonged effect is required**
WHAT	Liquid soap (e.g. Deb)	Skin disinfectants: • Alcohol hand rub (preferred) Skin disinfectants: • Chlorhexidine (e.g. Hibiscrub) • Povidone–Iodine (e.g. Betadine) Alcohol hand rub	• Chlorhexidine (e.g. Hibiscrub) • Povidone–Iodine (e.g. Betadine)
HOW	A thorough wash with cosmetically acceptable liquid soap	A thorough wash using six-step technique for 15–30 seconds or use alcohol hand rub following six-step technique	• Apply antiseptic soap to hands and forearms using a defined technique for a minimum of 2 minutes Alternatively: • Clean hands and forearms with soap and water • Apply 2 applications of an alcohol hand rub

WHEN

- Before and after performing routine tasks in all clinical areas
- During outbreaks of infection
- In high-risk areas
- When contact with infectious material is likely
- At the discretion of the infection control team
- Prior to surgery or invasive procedures

First aid following sharps/needle stick and splash incidents

Immediate action

- Encourage bleeding of wound
- Wash well with soap under running water and cover with waterproof dressing
- If body fluids splash into the mouth **do not** swallow, rinse out mouth several times with cold water. If into eyes, irrigate well with running water
- Report the incident to the senior person on duty in your area. Following exposure to known HIV contact senior nurse/duty manager
- Fill in an incident form
- Fill in the accident book

Ask yourself why the accident happened and what you can do to avoid a similar thing occurring again and discuss with your manager and colleagues. If you have not already considered having hepatitis B vaccine, think hard about it NOW!

CHAPTER 15

Common emergency treatments

Introduction

You will see patients being treated. The following notes provide a guide to the therapies that are employed. In each case a diagnosis needs to be made. The treatments apply to many situations. The specific causes may require additional therapy. These therapies were appropriate in May 2008, but with time, other therapies may become more appropriate.

Cardiovascular

Myocardial infarction (classic crushing, central chest pain with radiation to arms, pallor, sweating, distressed ± electrocardiogram (ECG) changes)

- Give 100% oxygen.
- Chew an aspirin—300 mg.
- Give diamorphine intravenously (i.v.) 2.5–5.0 mg or morphine i.v. 5.0–10.0 mg (±anti-emetic if necessary).
- Attach ECG monitor.
- If ST ≥2 mm new elevation in two or more contiguous chest leads or = 1 mm in standard leads or left bundle-branch block (LBBB):
    - institute thrombolysis with streptokinase, e.g. i.v. 1 500 000 U over 1 hour or tissue plasminogen activator (tPA) if no contraindication, e.g. bleeding, active peptic ulceration, recent

Clinical Skills and Examination: The Core Curriculum. By R Turner, B Angus, A Handa, C Hatton. ©2009 Blackwell Publishing, ISBN: 9781405157513.

operation, recent cerebral bleed or transient ischaemic attack, aortic aneurysm
    - hydrocortisone i.v. 100 mg if allergic reaction to streptokinase.
- If normal blood pressure (BP), well-perfused (warm hands), no heart failure give i.v. β-blocker, e.g. metoprolol 50 mg.
- If systolic BP <90 mmHg, periphery cold, monitor central venous pressure (CVP). Consider 250 ml 0.9 g/dl sodium chloride bolus. If continued hypotension and increasing CVP then seek help from intensive care for inotropic support.
- Treat arrhythmias (see Resuscitation Council guidelines, www.resus.org.uk).
- If left ventricular failure (crepitations, third heart sound, X-ray evidence) give furosemide 80 mg i.v. and consider intravenous nitrates and ACE inhibitors if systolic blood pressure above 100 mmHg.
- If urine output <30 ml/min, treat as acute renal failure (see below).
- After tPA give i.v. heparin.
- If at 24 hours BP >100 mmHg and no contraindication for oral β-blockers:
    - consider oral angiotensin-converting enzyme (ACE) inhibitors if anterior myocardial infarction, previous large myocardial infarction and heart failure
    - consider antihyperlipidaemic agents.

Acute coronary syndrome (continued myocardial pain without evidence of infarction)

- Give 100% oxygen.
- Chew an aspirin (300 mg); buccal GTN.
- Give subcutaneous low molecular heparin.
- Diamorphine + antiemetic.
- Consider GTN infusion i.v. starting at 1 mg/h, increase up to 10 mg/h as required—keep BP >100 mmHg.

- β-blocker orally if no clinical evidence of heart failure.
- Calcium antagonist orally, amlodipine if LVF poor or diltiazem if good LVF.
- Consider percutaneous transluminal coronary angioplasty (PTCA) either with balloon or stent angioplasty or coronary artery bypass graft (CABG) if pain does not settle (85% will settle on medical treatment).
- Consider antihyperlipidaemic agents such as a statin.

Acute left ventricular failure (breathless, tachycardia, triple rhythm, crepitations)

- Sit patient up.
- Give 100% oxygen.
- Attach ECG monitor and look for arrhythmias.
- Give i.v. 40–120 mg furosemide or i.v. 1–2 mg bumetanide.
- Give diamorphine i.v. 2.5–5.0 mg or morphine i.v. 5–10 mg (+an antiemetic e.g. i.v. 50 mg cyclizine or prochlorperazine 12.5 mg).
- If ventricular failure persists, consider ACE inhibitor or i.v. nitrate infusion.
- May require continuous positive airway pressure (CPAP) ventilation if no improvement and still dyspnoeic.

Arrhythmia

- **Bradycardia:** <40 beats/min, light-headed, black-outs, funny turns. Consider atropine 0.6 mg i.v. (repeat to max of 3 mg) or isoprenaline i.v. while waiting for pacemaker (see Resuscitation Council algorithm).
- **Tachycardia:** >140 beats/min in compromised patients, e.g. hypotension, heart failure, known heart disease (see Resuscitation Council algorithm).
  - Narrow-complex:
    - patient shocked: consider DC cardioversion
    - adenosine i.v. 3 mg
      then i.v. 6 mg if necessary
      then i.v. 12 mg if necessary

    - then i.v. amiodarone 300 mg in 30 minutes if necessary
    - verapamil i.v. may be used as an alternative (but not with β-blockers).
  - Broad-complex:
    - patient shocked: consider DC cardioversion
    - patient comfortable: i.v. amiodarone 300 mg in 30 minutes if necessary.
- **Ventricular fibrillation:** see Cardiac arrest instructions (see Resuscitation Council algorithm).

Severe hypertension (e.g. more than 220/120 mmHg, particularly if symptoms such as headaches or papilloedema)

- Recheck BP, with arterial line and continuous pressure monitoring, if available.
- Bring BP down over 24 hours (rapid reduction contraindicated as it can induce cerebral ischaemia).
- Use i.v. isosorbide mononitrate with monitoring.
- Or short acting oral β-blockers, ACE inhibitors or Ca^{2+} channel blocker (but not sublingual nifedipine).
- Treat any complications, e.g. left ventricular failure, encephalopathy.

Respiratory

Acute bronchospasm (breathless, wheeze, distress)

- Give 100% oxygen unless known chronic airways disease (see below).
- Salbutamol by nebulizer (not inhalers) 5 ml in 2 ml water.
- Hydrocortisone 100 mg i.v. and oral prednisolone 30–50 mg.
- If necessary intravenous magnesium
- **If necessary** aminophylline 5 mg/kg i.v. by slow injection (10–15 minutes) with cardiac monitoring but **not** if patient has taken theophyllines already.
- Do blood gases:

	Po_2 (in pKa)	Pco_2 (in pKa)
• Mild	<10	<4
• Moderate	8–10	<4
• Severe	<8	4–6: watch carefully
• Desperate	<7	>6: consider ventilation

- Monitor fatigue—consider ventilation if patient becomes exhausted. Remember to let intensive care know sooner rather than later.

Acute exacerbation in chronic obstructive airways disease (usually breathless, cough, sputum and coarse crepitations)

- Give 24% oxygen and increase if $P\text{CO}_2$ not raised.
- Blood gases:
  - P_{O_2}¬ and P_{CO_2} ↓ '**pink puffer**': increase oxygen content
  - P_{O_2}¬ and P_{CO_2} ↑ '**blue bloater**': increase oxygen carefully, repeating blood gases, as removal of hypoxic drive may decrease respiratory volume and rate. Then reduce P_{O_2} and consider doxapram. Ventilation may be indicated when there is a good prognosis
- Physiotherapy to cough up sputum.
- Chest X-ray, consider oral antibiotics such as doxycycline.

Gastrointestinal

Acute gastrointestinal haemorrhage (sudden collapse, haematemesis or red/black sticky stools; BP <100 mmHg, pulse >100 beats/min). Use Rockall score (see Appendix 7).

- Assess whether cirrhosis/portal hypertension, peptic ulcer.
- Establish i.v. access (two large venflons) and take blood for haematology, biochemistry and crossmatching.
- If BP <90 mmHg, 500 ml 0.9 g/dl sodium chloride or colloid in 30 minutes.
- If no BP, consider group O rhesus-negative blood.

- If no central pulse, for cardiorespiratory resuscitation.
- Monitor CVP.
- Give blood as required to raise BP and CVP.
- Urinary catheter if severe blood loss.
- Alert surgical team and arrange urgent endoscopy.

Acute hepatic failure (jaundice, foetor, liver flap, confusion)

- If systolic BP <90 mmHg, 500 ml i.v. 5% dextrose or colloid in 30 minutes.
- Monitor CVP.
- Monitor blood glucose—if <4 mmol/l, infuse dextrose 10% and recheck.
- Look for drugs, including paracetamol overdose.
- Look for infection—blood, chest, urine, ascites.
- Look for occult bleeding, including increasing plasma urea:
  - consider fresh frozen plasma to correct clotting.
- Start oral lactulose.
- Prevent stress ulcers with H_2-blocker or proton pump blocker.
- Vitamins B and K i.v.
- Restrict salt and water intake.
- Monitor drugs, electrolyte, liver function tests, clotting, pH.

Neurological

Epileptic attack (tonic/clonic movements, usually unconscious)

- Oxygen.
- Bedside test for glucose—?hypoglycaemia.
- Diazepam or lorazepam pr or i.v. 5–10 mg over 2 minutes, then i.v. 2 mg/min for 20 minutes or until fit ceases. Watch for respiratory depression.
- Phenytoin i.v. 50 mg/min.
- If fit continues:
  - chlormethiazole or phenytoin
  - general anaesthesia and ventilate.

Unconsciousness with no overt cause

- Clear airway and give 100% oxygen.
- Prone recovery position unless airway protected by endotracheal tube.
- Examine for head injury, neurological deficit, neck stiffness.
- Enquire whether diabetic or access to insulin, any tablets or whether a suicide risk.
- Prevent fitting (see above).
- If respiratory rate <10 breaths/min give i.v. naloxone.
- Check blood glucose.
- If BP <90 mmHg systolic, give 500 ml 0.9 g/dl sodium chloride or colloid i.v.
- Check blood gases.
- Take blood and urine for drug tests.
- Document level of consciousness on Glasgow Coma Scale.

Meningitis (headache, neck stiffness, vomiting, photophobia, febrile)

- **N.B.** if purpuric rash, immediately start i.v. antibiotic—ceftriaxone 2 g—after taking blood cultures.
- Check for signs of raised intracranial pressure, e.g. papilloedema.
- Lumbar puncture safe if no signs of raised intracranial pressure but usually wait for CT after giving antibiotics:
  - note pressure
  - cerebrospinal fluid (CSF) for culture—bacterial, PCR for viruses, biochemistry and microscopy.
- Cloudy CSF (white cells)—prompt i.v. antibiotics after blood cultures.
- Blood-stained—assess whether bloody tap, i.e. blood at first then clearing, or subarachnoid haemorrhage (consistent blood with xanthochromia of CSF after centrifuging down red cells).

Other systems

Acute renal failure (rapid increase in plasma creatinine, urine output <30 ml/h)

- Consider **prerenal** cause (patient 'dehydrated'—dry tongue, low skin turgor, empty veins, low CVP, low blood pressure)—give fluid challenge and continue until JVP is 2–3 cm above the manubriosternal junction.
- Consider **postrenal** cause (e.g. enlarged prostate, bilateral ureteric stones, renal/pelviureteric obstruction). If large prostate and large bladder, consider passing catheter.
- If no obvious cause of renal failure, ultrasound abdomen—?dilated ureters or dilated renal pelves or small kidneys, indicating chronic renal failure.
- Check plasma potassium, sodium, creatinine, urea (if potassium >6 mmol/l and ECG changes, give i.v. glucose/insulin, i.v. calcium gluconate and rectal cation exchange resin).
- Check urine sodium and osmolality
  - in prerenal failure, urine osmolality >400 mosmol/kg and sodium <30 mmol/l
  - in renal failure, <400 mosmol/kg and >30 mmol/l, respectively.
- Microscope urine sediment for red cells, white cells, casts and bacteria.
- Check arterial pH.
- When fluid-replete, restrict fluid to 500 ml per day + previous day's losses.
- High-energy, low-protein diet.
- Watch for infection.
- Consider dialysis if creatinine >400 μmol/l or potassium remains >6 mmol/l, fluid overload, acidosis or pericarditis.

Diabetic ketoacidosis (usually known diabetic patient; ketoacidosis induced by infection, vomiting, missing insulin injections; patient is drowsy, 'dehydrated' ± ketotic breath)

- Check plasma glucose, electrolytes, arterial pH, CRP, troponin, blood and urine culture, ECG and chest X-ray.
- Check urine for ketones; measure in ketone meter if possible, otherwise use serum or urinary ketones. If there are no ketones consider hyperosmolar, non-ketotic coma.
- Fluid replacement—initially N saline—typically 1 litre over 30 mins, 1 litre over 2 h, 1 litre over 4 h, 1 litre over 6 h then 8-hourly. When glucose levels are less than 1 litre mmol/l switch to 5% dextrose. (Remember this would need to be modified with co-morbidity, e.g. CCF)
  - CVP line to assess volume requirement may be necessary.
- Stat dose of insulin 10 units actrapid i.m.
- Insulin infusion (50 units actrapid in 50 ml of N saline to run i.v. according to sliding scale): aim to reduce glucose level by 6 mmol/h.

Sliding scale:

Glucose (mmol/l)	Insulin (U/hour)
>20	6
17–20	5
14–17	4
11–14	3
7–10	2
4–7	1
<4	0.5

- Measure ketones and glucose hourly and adjust insulin accordingly.
- If very drowsy, nasogastric tube to prevent inhalation of vomit.
- Potassium replacement—none if K^+ <5.5 mmol/l. Otherwise, add potassium 20–40 mmol/l to each litre of i.v. saline.

Hypoglycaemia (symptoms include drowsy/unconscious, perspiring, tachycardia, bounding pulse, usually in insulin-treated diabetic due to missing snack or increased exercise. N.B. many diabetic patients are asymptomatic with hypoglycaemia)

- Check plasma glucose. (Do not await result from laboratory—treat straight away.)
- Keep airway clear.
- If no i.v. access give 1 mg glucagon i.m., acts in 5–10 minutes (but not if hypoglycaemia due to insulinoma).
- If emergency, e.g. fitting, 50 ml 50 g/dl i.v. glucose followed by 50 ml of 0.9 g/dl saline to wash sclerosant, hypertonic glucose out of vein.

Septicaemia (febrile >39°C, rigors)

- Give 100% oxygen.
- Look for source of septicaemia including skin, chest, urine, abdomen and meningitis.
- If systolic BP <90 mmHg, 500 ml i.v. sodium chloride or colloid i.v. in 30 minutes.
- Monitor CVP.
- Antibiotics i.v. after blood cultures, culture of urine, throat or pustules.
- If neutropenic sepsis give empirical antibiotics usually antipseudomonal penicillin, e.g. meropenem or piperacillin/tazobactam plus aminoglycoside, e.g. gentamicin.
- If BP ↓, pH ↓ or consciousness level ↓—transfer to intensive care unit.

Poisoning or overdose

- Give 100% oxygen, except in paraquat poisoning.
- Check paracetamol and aspirin levels in all patients.
- Give naloxone if respiratory rate <10 breaths/min. Measure blood gases and consider ventilation.
- Correct hypotension: if BP <90 mmHg, 500 ml i.v. sodium chloride in 30 minutes.
- Consider gastric lavage—intubate first if unconscious.
- Paracetamol overdose—acetylcysteine according to blood levels of paracetamol.

- Aspirin overdose:
  - gastric lavage up to 12 hours
  - watch pH
  - consider forced alkaline diuresis.
- Amphetamine poisoning:
  - beware sudden airway oedema
  - have available intubation equipment, adrenaline, chlorpheniramine, hydrocortisone.
- Consider activated charcoal per oral/gastric tube.
- If potentially an unusual poison, phone poison centre for advice.

Anaphylactic response

- Give 100% oxygen.
- Chlorpheniramine 10 mg i.v. in 1 minute.
- Hydrocortisone 100 mg i.v.
- If severe, adrenaline 0.5–1 mg i.v. slowly over 1–2 minutes.
- If BP <90 mmHg, 500 ml i.v. sodium chloride or colloid.

Death

While a diagnosis of death *per se* does not require emergency therapy, the required procedures are an important aspect of medicine.

If there is sudden loss of consciousness, consider cardiopulmonary resuscitation—see Cardiac arrest instructions (Appendix 3).

- Pale, pulseless, apnoeic—listen at mouth, observe chest.
- No heart sounds—listen with diaphragm.
- Fixed pupils.
- Head and eyes move together when head moved, i.e. no oculocephalic reflex movement or 'doll's eye' movement.
- No corneal response.
- No response to any stimulus.

If the patient is cold, <35°C, or there has been a major drug overdose, e.g. barbiturate, they can appear dead.

If in doubt look at retina with ophthalmoscope to see if 'trucking' of non-flowing segments of blood in veins.

Brain death criteria

- If the patient is on a ventilator because of apnoea, test:
  - at least 6 hours after onset of coma
  - at least 24 hours after cardiac arrest/circulation restoration
  - by two independent consultants if feasible.
- Whether patient has condition that could lead to irremediable brain damage.
- There are no reflex responses or epileptic jerks.
- No hypothermia—temperature >35°C.
- No drug intoxication—off therapy for 48 hours
  - particularly depressants, neuromuscular-blocking (relaxant) drugs.
- No hypoglycaemia, acidosis, gross electrolyte imbalance.
- All brainstem reflexes absent, confirmed by two physicians:
  - no pupil response to light.
- No corneal reflexes.
- No vestibular-ocular reflexes:
  - visualise tympanic membranes
  - 20 ml cold water in each ear
  - no eye movements.
- No cranial motor responses:
  - no gag reflex
  - no cough reflex to bronchial stimulaton.
- No respiratory effort when ventilator is stopped:
  - P_{CO_2} rise to 6.7 kPa.
- Repeat tests at least 2 hours later, usually after 24 hours.
- Time of second test is legally the time of death.

N.B. Spinal reflexes and electroencephalogram are irrelevant. Warn family that reflex leg movements can exist after cessation of brainstem function and are not of relevance.

Appendices

Appendix 1: Jaeger reading chart

Jaeger types assess visual acuity for close tasks. They provide the easiest quick method of assessment. The patient should use their spectacles normally required for reading. Ask the patient to read the smallest type they can read, if read with few mistakes, ask them to read the next size down. Record the size of type that can be read with each eye separately.

Appendix 2: Visual acuity 3 m chart

The 3-m Snellen chart should be held at 3 m from the patient, with good lighting, with each of the patient's eyes covered in turn. Use the patient's usual spectacles for this distance. If the patient cannot read 6/6 (e.g. 6/12 is best vision in one eye), repeat without spectacles and with a 'pinhole' that largely nullifies refractive errors. Note for each eye the best acuity obtained and the method used, e.g. L 6/9 R 6/6 with spectacles.

V H

36

X U A

24

H T Y O

18

V U A X T

12

H A Y O U X

9

Y U X T H A O V

6

X O A T V H U Y

5

Appendix 3: Cardiac arrest instructions

Resuscitation Council (UK)

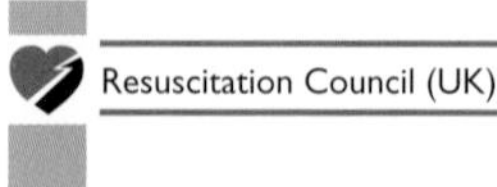

Adult Basic Life Support

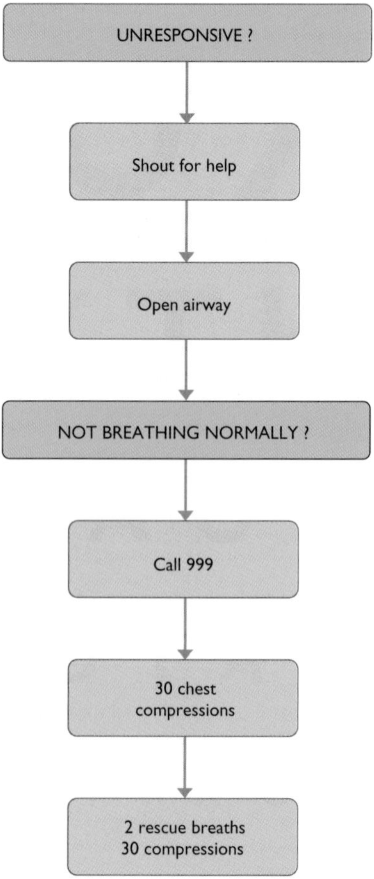
UNRESPONSIVE ?
Shout for help
Open airway
NOT BREATHING NORMALLY ?
Call 999
30 chest compressions
2 rescue breaths
30 compressions

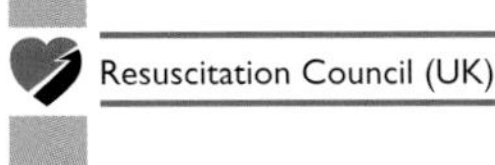

Adult Advanced Life Support Algorithm

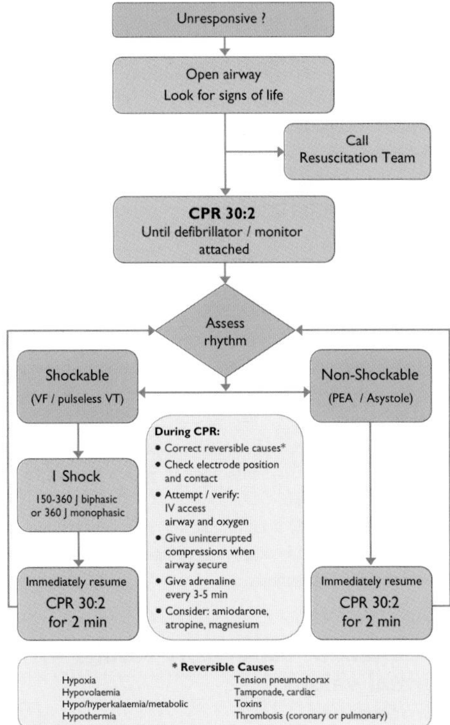

Appendix 4: Duties of a doctor

General Medical Council (2006) guidelines state:

The duties of a doctor registered with the General Medical Council

Patients must be able to trust doctors with their lives and health. To justify that trust you must show respect for human life and you must:

Make the care of your patient your first concern
Protect and promote the health of patients and the public
Provide a good standard of practice and care
Keep your professional knowledge and skills up to date
Recognise and work within the limits of your competence
Work with colleagues in the ways that best serve patients' interests
Treat patients as individuals and respect their dignity
Treat patients politely and considerately
Respect patients' right to confidentiality
Work in partnership with patients
Listen to patients and respond to their concerns and preferences
Give patients the information they want or need in a way they can understand
Respect patients' right to reach decisions with you about their treatment and care
Support patients in caring for themselves to improve and maintain their health
Be honest and open and act with integrity
Act without delay if you have good reason to believe that you or a colleague may be putting patients at risk
Never discriminate unfairly against patients or colleagues
Never abuse your patients' trust in you or the public's trust in the profession
You are personally accountable for your professional practice and must always be prepared to justify your decisions and actions.

Appendix 5: Laboratory results—normal values

Introduction

Normal ranges are the most frequently used reference interval. For some situations, **specific diagnostic reference intervals** are appropriate, e.g. twice normal value of plasma creatine kinase for diagnosing Duchenne muscular dystrophy.

Action limits can be set which aid decision taking, e.g. a cholesterol value in the upper normal range (>6.5 mmol/l) may require therapy.

Patient-specific reference intervals are sometimes required for therapeutic purposes, e.g. specific glucose control criteria for different diabetic patients.

Methods and their normal ranges vary from laboratory to laboratory and according to the sex and age distribution of the reference healthy population. The following results are a general guide for adults' values and may not be apposite for your laboratory.

Haematology

	Male	Female
Haemoglobin	13.5–18.0 g/dl	11.5–16.0 g/dl
Packed cell volume (PCV)	40–54%	37–47%
Red cell count	4.5–6.5 ∞ 10^{12}/l	3.9–5.6 ∞ 10^{12}/l
Mean cell volume (MCV)	76–100 fl	
Mean cell haemoglobin	27–32 pg	
Mean cell haemoglobin concentration	32–36 g/dl	
Reticulocyte count	0.8–2%	
White cell count	4.0–11.0 × 10^9/l	
Platelets	150–450 × 10^9/l	
Prothrombin time	10–14 s	
Activated partial thromboplastin time	30–40 s	
INR therapeutic range for treatment of DVT	2.0–3.0	
Erythrocyte sedimentation rate (ESR) Westergren at 1 hour	0–10 mm (higher values of ESR may occur in normal elderly patients)	0–15 mm

Cerebrospinal fluid

Cells	0–5 white cells
	0 red cells
Glucose	2.8–4.2 mmol/l
Pressure	70–180 mmH_2O
Protein	0.15–0.45 g/l

Clinical chemistry (in SI units)

Serum or plasma

ACE (angiotensin-converting enzyme)	20–54 U/l
Acid phosphatase (total)	1–5 iu/l
Acid phosphatase (prostatic)	0–1 iu/l
ACTH (adrenocorticotrophic hormone)	<80 μg/l
Albumin	35–50 g/l
Aldosterone, recumbent (doubles after 30 min in upright posture)	100–500 pmol/l
Alkaline phosphatase (adult)	80–250 iu/l
Alpha-1antitrypsin	107–209 mg/dl
Amylase	25–180 Somogyi units/dl
Anion gap	7–16 mmol/l
Aspartate aminotransferase (AST)	15–42 iu/l
Bicarbonate	24–30 mmol/l
Bilirubin (total)	3–17 μmol/l
Bilirubin in babies (toxic value)	>300 μmol/l
Bilirubin (conjugated)	0–5 μmol/l
C-peptide (fasting—interpret with glucose value)	0.2–0.8 nmol/l
C-reactive protein	<10 mg/l
Caeruloplasmin	16–60 mg/dl
Calcitonin	<0.08 μg/l
Calcium (with normal albumin level)	2.12–2.65 mmol/l
Carbon monoxide—non-smoker	0–2%

Carbon monoxide—smoker	up to 5%
Carcinoembryonic antigen (CEA)	0–9 μmol/l
Catecholamines	
–noradrenaline	<5.7 μmol/l
–adrenaline	<2.1 μmol/l
Chloride	95–105 mmol/l
Cholesterol (population reference)	3.9–7.8 mmol/l
Copper	12–26 μmol/l
Cortisol (0900 h)	280–700 nmol/l
Cortisol (midnight)	80–280 nmol/l
Creatine kinase (women)	24–195 iu/l
Creatine kinase (men)	24–170 iu/l
Creatinine	70–150 μmol/l
11-Deoxycortisol	7–16 nmol/l
DHEAS (dehydroepiandrosterone sulphate) (women)	4.9–9.4 μmol/l
DHEAS (men)	2.3–12.0 μmol/l
Ferritin (women)	15–140 μg/l
Ferritin (men)	17–230 μg/l
α-Fetoprotein (AFP)	0–14 kU/l
Folate (serum)	2.1–18 μg/l
Folate (red cell)	160–640 μg/l
Follicle-stimulating hormone (female luteal)	2–8 U/l
Follicle-stimulating hormone (postmenopausal women)	>30 U/l
Follicle-stimulating hormone (men)	0.5–5.0 U/l
Gastrin (fasting)	<40 pmol/l
Gastro-inhibitory peptide (fasting)	<300 pmol/l
Glucagon (fasting)	<50 pmol/l
Glucose (plasma, fasting)	3.8–5.5 mmol/l
γ-Glutamyl transpeptidase (women)	7–40 iu/l
γ-Glutamyl transpeptidase (men)	11–51 iu/l

Haemoglobin A_{1c}	4.5–6.2%
HDL (high density lipoprotein) cholesterol	0.8–2.0 mmol/l
Human chorionic gonadotrophin (HCG)	0–5 iu/l
17α-Hydroxyprogesterone	<20 nmol/l
Immunoglobulin A	0.8–3.0 g/l
Immunoglobulin E	<80 kU/l
Immunoglobulin G	6.0–13.0 g/l
Immunoglobulin M	0.4–2.5 g/l
Insulin (fasting—interpret with glucose value)	2–13 mU/l
Iron (women)	11–30 μmol/l
Iron (men)	14–31 μmol/l
Iron-binding capacity	45–70 μmol/l
Lactate (fasting)	0.6–2.0 mmol/l
Lactate dehydrogenase	110–250 iu/l
Lead (blood)	<0.7 μmol/l
Luteinizing hormone (female luteal)	3–6 U/l
Luteinizing hormone (postmenopausal women)	>30 U/l
Luteinizing hormone (men)	3–8 U/l
Magnesium	0.75–1.05 mmol/l
17β-Oestradiol (female luteal)	180–1100 pmol/l
17β-Oestradiol (men)	<220 pmol/l
Osmolality	278–305 mosmol/kg
Parathyroid hormone (PTH)	0.9–5.4 pmol/l
Phosphate	0.8–1.45 mmol/l
Potassium	3.5–5.0 mmol/l
Progesterone (female luteal)	16–77 nmol/l
Progesterone (men)	0–6 nmol/l
Prolactin (women)	<450 mU/l
Prolactin (men)	<400 mU/l
Prostate-specific antigen (PSA)	<4 μg/l
Protein (total)	60–80 g/l
Pyruvate	41–67 μmol/
Renin (recumbent)	1.1–2.7 pmol/ml/h
Renin (erect)	2.8–4.5 pmol/ml/h

Sodium	134–145 mmol/l
Testosterone (women)	1.0–2.5 nmol/l
Testosterone (men)	9–42 nmol/l
Thyroxine	70–140 nmol/l
Thyroxine (free)	9–25 pmol/l
Transaminase (GOT, AST)	5–35 iu/l
Transaminase (GPT, ALT)	5–45 iu/l
Triglyceride (fasting)	0.6–1.9 mmol/l
Triiodothyronine	1.0–3.0 nmol/l
Triiodothyronine (free)	3.4–7.2 pmol/l
TSH (thyroid-stimulating hormone)	0.5–6.0 mU/l
Urate (women)	150–390 μmol/l
Urate (men)	210–480 μmol/l
Urea	2.5–6.7 mmol/l
VIP (vasoactive intestinal polypeptide)	<30 pmol/l
Vitamin B_{12}	150–750 ng/l
Vitamin D	7–50 μg/l
Vitamin E	11.5–35.0 μmol/l
Zinc	6–25 μmol/l

24-hour urine

Aldosterone	10–50 nmol/day
δ-Amino laevulinic acid	9.5–53.4 μmol/day
Calcium	2.5–7.5 mmol/day
Chloride	110–250 mmol/day
Copper	0.2–1.0 μmol/day
Coproporphyrin	51–350 nmol/day
Cortisol	28–280 nmol/day
Creatinine clearance (women)	85–125 ml/min
Creatinine clearance (men)	95–140 ml/min
5-HIAA (5-OH indoleacetic acid)	10.4–41.6 μmol/day
Homovanillic acid (HVA)	<82 μmol/day
Metadrenaline	<2 μmol/day
Normetadrenaline	<3 μmol/day
OH methylmandelic acid (HMMA)	10–35 μmol/day

Osmolality	50–1400 mOsmol/kg
Osmolality (after 12 h fluid restriction)	>850 mOsmol/kg
pH	5.5–8.0 pH units
Phosphate	12.9–42 mmol/day
Porphobilinogen	0–10 μmol/day
Potassium	40–120 mmol/day
Protein	50–80 mg/day
Sodium	60–280 mmol/day
Urea	164–600 mmol/day

Drugs in serum

The following are usual therapeutic ranges. The value related to the time of ingestion is crucial for some drugs, e.g. plasma paracetamol >1.0 mmol/l gives a risk of liver damage but the decision interval of the plasma level for therapy decreases with time after an overdose.

Amiodarone—before dose	0.6–2.0 mg/l
Carbamazepine—before dose	34–51 μmol/l
Carbamazepine (children)	17–35 μmol/l
Carbon monoxide—non-smoker	0–2%
Carbon monoxide—smoker	0–5%
Clonazepam—before dose	25–85 μg/l
Digoxin—at least 6 hours after last dose	1.0–2.0 nmol/l
Disopyramide—before dose	2.0–5.0 mg/dl
Epanutin—before dose	40–80 μmol/l
Ethosuximide—before dose	40–80 mg/l
Lithium	0.5–1.5 mmol/l
Phenobarbitone—before dose	65–170 μmol/l
Phenytoin—before dose	40–80 μmol/l
Salicylate	0.4–2.5 mmol/l
Theophylline—before dose	55–110 μmol/l
Valproate—before dose	0.3–0.7 mmol/l

Toxic levels

Barbiturate—potentially fatal	
• short-acting	35 μmol/l
• medium-acting	105 μmol/l
• long-acting	215 μmol/l
Ethanol (physiological <0.2 nmol/l)	
• legal limit for driving	<17.4 nmol/l
Paracetamol—risk of liver damage	
• at 4 hours	>1.32 mmol/l
• at 15 hours	<0.2 mmol/l
Salicylate	>2.5 mmol/l

Miscellaneous

Faecal fat	<18 mmol/day
Sweat chloride	6–40 mmol/l
Extractable nuclear antigen-binding	association
Anti-Ro	SLE, cutaneous lupus
Anti-La	SLE, Sjögren's disease
Anti-Sm	SLE (specific)
Anti-RNP	SLE, mixed connective tissue disease
Anti-Scl-70	Progressive systemic sclerosis
Anti-Jo 1	Polymyositis

Appendix 6: Examples of OSCE assessment stations

- Abdominal X-ray
- Chest X-ray
- ECG interpretation
- Abdominal examination
- Resuscitation (basic life support)
- History of a core surgical complaint
- History of a core medical complaint
- Peripheral pulse examination
- Neck examination
- Breast examination
- Interpretation of results e.g. ECG, urinalysis, arterial blood gases

- Interpretation of results e.g. full blood count, liver function tests, urea and creatinine, other biochemistry
- Interpretation of patient observation charts, e.g. fluid balance, TPR chart, peak flow charts, blood glucose
- Practical procedures, e.g. phlebotomy, NG tube insertion, arterial blood gas, ECG, IV line insertion
- Examination of lumps
- General examination of a patient
- Cardiovascular examination
- Respiratory examination
- Cranial nerve/peripheral nerve examination

Appendix 7: Rockall score

	Rockall score			
Variable	0	1	2	3
Age	<60	60–79	>80	
Shock	No shock	Pulse >100	SBP <100	
Comorbidity	Nil major		CCF, IHD, major morbidity	Renal failure, liver failure, metastatic cancer
Diagnosis	Likely diagnosis Mallory-Weiss	All other diagnoses	GI malignancy	
Evidence of bleeding	None	Blood	Blood, adherent clot	Spurting vess

Interpretation

Total score is calculated by simple addition. A score of less than 3 carries a good prognosis but a total score more than 8 carries high risk of mortality.

Index